Penguin Handbooks

VOGUE GUIDE TO SKIN CARE

Felicity Clark has been Beauty Editor of *Vogue* since 1972. She started her career in public relations and later worked for five years in New York as executive assistant to Diana Vreeland, then editor-in-chief of American *Vogue*. She joined Condé Nast in London in 1969.

As the daughter of a regular army officer, she travelled a lot as a child – and has continued doing so in her job. She is an active sportswoman and a gifted musician – she played the flute in the National Youth Orchestra.

She has worked with leading photographers all over the world. Lord Snowdon says: 'She is one of the most professional editors that I have ever worked with. There are many assignments that I would not have been able to do without her tremendous contribution. It is the back-up that she supplies, the amount of research and meticulous attention to detail that she puts in beforehand. On the assignment itself, she manages to create an atmosphere that stimulates and encourages everyone involved.'

VOGUE GUIDE
TO SKIN CARE

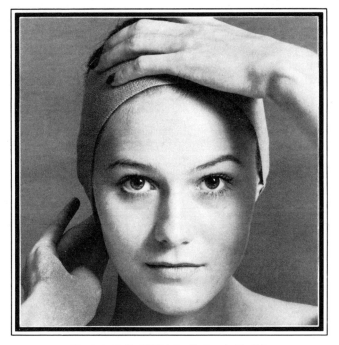

FELICITY CLARK

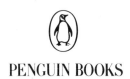

PENGUIN BOOKS

Penguin Books Ltd, Harmondsworth, Middlesex, England
Penguin Books, 625 Madison Avenue, New York, New York 10022, U.S.A.
Penguin Books Australia Ltd, Ringwood, Victoria, Australia
Penguin Books Canada Ltd, 2801 John Street, Markham, Ontario, Canada L3R 1B4
Penguin Books (N.Z.) Ltd, 182–190 Wairau Road, Auckland 10, New Zealand

First published 1981

Set in Monophoto Photina by Filmtype Services Limited, Scarborough, Yorks
Made and printed in Great Britain by Butler & Tanner Ltd, Frome and London

Designed by Patrick Yapp

Contents

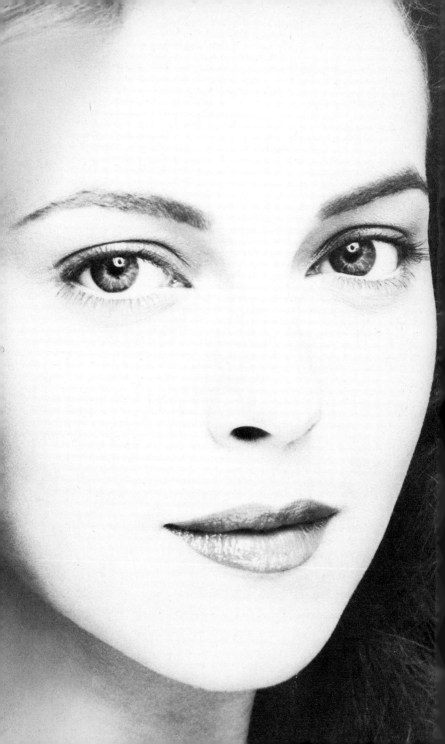

Introduction

The purpose of this guide is to help you understand your skin and help it to look its best by making sure you know what affects it well and badly, what kind of products to choose, what to avoid. After all, it is one of the body's main organs (taking up a very large proportion of the visible area) and accounts for one twentieth of its weight. Did you know it gathers supplies, gets rid of waste, manufactures lubricants, feeds growing hairs, nourishes nails on fingers and toes? It is working extremely hard all the time and deserves every bit of help you can give it.

Skin is one of the few tissues that replenishes itself, constantly shedding dead cells and producing new ones. It is this that provides its texture and fresh look. And, it is a slowing-down of this process that causes it to lose its elasticity and colour and look old. It starts to slow down almost from the moment we are born. The skin of a new-born baby is much admired and often used as a yardstick when comparing skin. This, of course, is the newest, softest and purest we know; and as we grow older, so does the skin. It coarsens and develops until we have our individual skin character – a type that may be oily, blemished, dry, sensitive, balanced or a combination; a texture that may be coarse, medium or fine; a colouring that is pale, medium or dark.

Everyday exposure to the elements (sun, wind, rain, extreme heat or cold) and, recently, the popularity of intensive sunbathing, sports like snow and water-skiing, the accumulation of pollution in the air around us – all have damaging effects on the skin.

It is obviously a tremendous beauty asset and has been admired since the earliest records – Cleopatra, for instance (one of the first celebrity beauties), was known to bathe in asses' milk, which she believed softened and improved her skin. (Even now many skin and bath products are called milks although, of course, they don't necessarily contain real milk.)

Slowing up the ageing process has been a major source of concern in the lives of beautiful women throughout history, and we are lucky enough to live in an era when science brings help within the reach of all women. Researchers into the mechanism of the human body are constantly making new discoveries in the world of health and medicine, and often new beauty aids are a spin-off.

So, much can be done to prolong the youth of your skin by keeping your body in top condition through exercise, diet and beauty routines. This guide aims to tell you about every inch of skin on your body, where it's most vulnerable, when it may need expert help, how to look after it day by day.

There are two companion books to this one – *Vogue Guide to Hair Care* and *Vogue Guide to Make-up*, also published by Penguin Books.

Helmut Newton

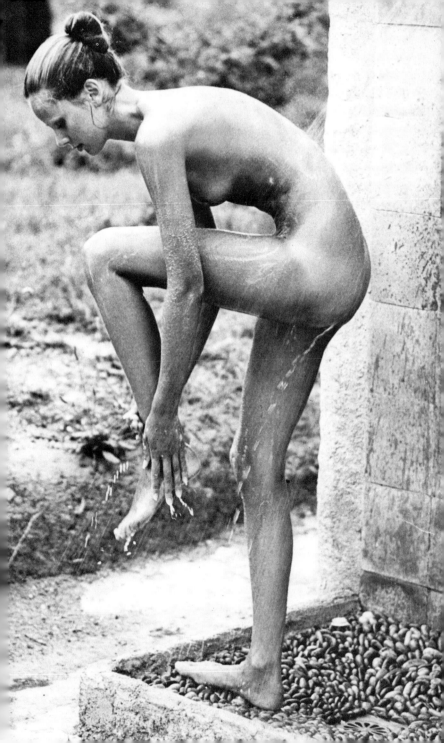

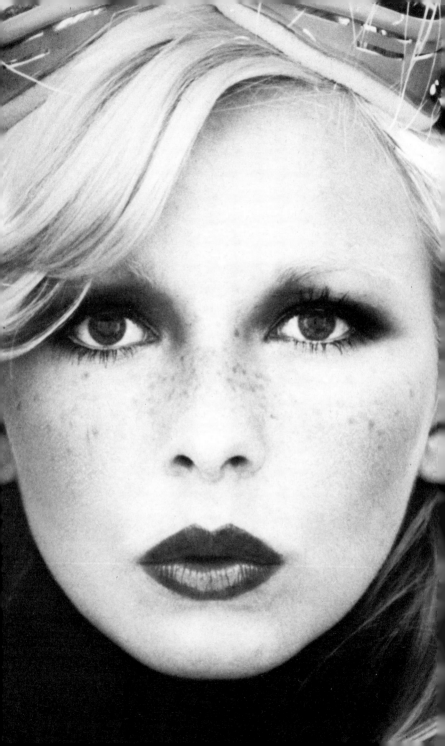

Skin:
What It Is and What It Does

Skin is a tissue covering the whole body – approximately one and a half square metres. It consists of areas called the *epidermis*, a visible surface layer with no blood-vessels; the *dermis*, full of collagen fibres, cells that store and release vital moisture, and nourishing blood-vessels; glands for lubrication (sebaceous) and for regulating body temperatures (sweat); and an important layer of fat that feeds the sebaceous glands and acts as a cushion between surface skin and muscle below. The epidermis, having no blood-vessels, will heal without trace. The dermis, on the other hand, if damaged, will result in scars: it is this layer, which is full of blood-vessels, that is affected by emotions and causes blushing and other changes in colour. Some people, for instance, turn white from panic or shock and this is caused by the draining-away of these blood-vessels; others turn green if they're feeling ill and this is a yellow bile from the liver coming to the surface through them. The glands function through the pores which are exit channels, visible to the eye and which, if the skin isn't cleaned properly, become clogged and form whiteheads or blackheads. It is the sebaceous glands which decide whether your skin is oily (they are over-active), dry (they are sluggish) or normal (they are functioning well). Beneath the scalp they will determine whether your hair is oily, dry or normal.

The depth and quality of your skin changes in different parts of the body. The scalp is densely populated with hair follicles fed by the sebaceous glands and needs to be kept scrupulously clean to avoid problems and encourage healthy hair. The face holds many variations – the eye area is more transparent and delicate than anywhere else; the lips, mouth and inner nose are entirely different, being moist mucous membrane (likewise the vaginal area); the neck tends to be dry. Areas of the body normally covered by clothing retain their natural softness longer than limbs and extremities like hands and feet. The skin on palms and soles is the thickest and toughest of all. Then, there are armpits, which hold sweat-glands and contain more hair follicles; breasts, which have a transparent quality all their own; the genital area, which also has its own sweat-glands and hair follicles; and the gluteal fold of the buttocks. Hormones are essential to the satisfactory functioning of the body and play a vital part in the skin's activity: they stimulate pigment cells and regulate colour; they affect the production of sebum (so necessary to healthy hair); the secretion of the adrenal glands stimulates the sweat-glands; hormones control the breasts, which often change during the menstrual cycle and swell before menstruation, giving the skin a stretched translucent appearance and a feeling of discomfort from the extra liquid. Hormonal imbalance can cause enlarged pores, which sometimes leads to acne.

Nerves, too, are an important area. Contact is made through the skin, giving sensations such as tickling, touch, temperature changes, itching, pain, taste, smell and sexual arousal. Nerves vary in density in different areas of the body and vary from person to person – hence, one person may be ticklish in the ribs or soles of the feet, another not.

A good diet, exercise, sleep, fresh air and plenty of water are necessary if your skin is to look its best. On the other hand, it will react badly to emotional stress and tension and it will suffer from sun and wind if not protected. Deodorant-antiperspirants should be used sparingly or glands will cease to function properly; also avoid excessive washing and beware of unqualified 'beauticians' in fields like massage and hair removal.

Lothar Schmid

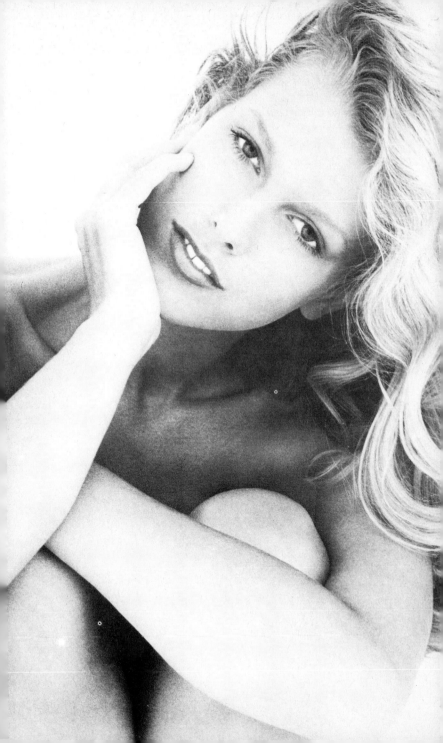

Skin Types:
Which Is Yours?

Your ancestors and immediate parentage, through your genes, will have determined your skin colour and the bone structure which gives faces their characteristics. Your skin may be pale, olive, or black – with variations on all three – and your race descends from one of the ancient world's main four: Caucasian, Negro, Mongolian and Australian. All these probably developed from a single origin and have interbred over the centuries, so the distinctive features of skull shape, hair type and skin colour have diminished and probably rarely exist now in pure form. Whatever your race, skin is usually divided into four types: oily, dry, a combination of the two and balanced, with two subsidiary categories, sensitive and blemished. The word 'healthy' in relation to skin means smooth skin that glows with colour, is free of blemishes and is clean. This is the kind of skin you should have, and once you have discovered your skin type, provided you stick to a regular correct skin-treatment routine (and the wonderful thing about skin is that it does respond to care and can be improved), it is the kind of skin you can have.

Oily Skin
Oily skin comes from over-active sebaceous glands. It shines excessively, tends to break out and is the most likely candidate to suffer from acne. If you have oily skin you will probably also find you have enlarged pores and oily hair; you are also likely to be under twenty, after which hormones are more stable and skin

often undergoes a change for the better. It is to your advantage that oily skin develops fewer wrinkles and stays looking younger longer.

Blemished Skin

Blemished skin usually results from oily skin which has suffered from spots and acne and, in the worst cases, scarred permanently. It can also be the result of diseases like chicken-pox and measles.

Dry Skin

Dry skin tends to flake and has a matt texture with little or no shine. It is the result of dehydration – the sebaceous glands are sluggish, or the skin has been over-exposed to sun, wind and central heating. This type of skin rarely suffers from spots, and pores are hardly visible, but the condition doesn't improve with age and wrinkles will appear early.

Sensitive Skin

Sensitive skin is usually a consequence of dry skin, is often allergic to many cosmetics, tends to develop red patches from broken capillaries near the skin's surface and cannot be exposed to direct sunlight. Certain foods, alcoholic drinks, stress and emotional problems may also affect this type.

Combination Skin

Combination skin usually has a T-shaped panel of oiliness down the centre (across the forehead and down the middle and sides of the nose and mouth), with dry areas on cheeks and towards the hairline.

Balanced Skin

Balanced skin is what everyone would like to possess, but few do. The skin will appear fine-textured, smooth and well-coloured, will rarely break out and will retain its youthful quality well, although it will probably become drier after thirty.

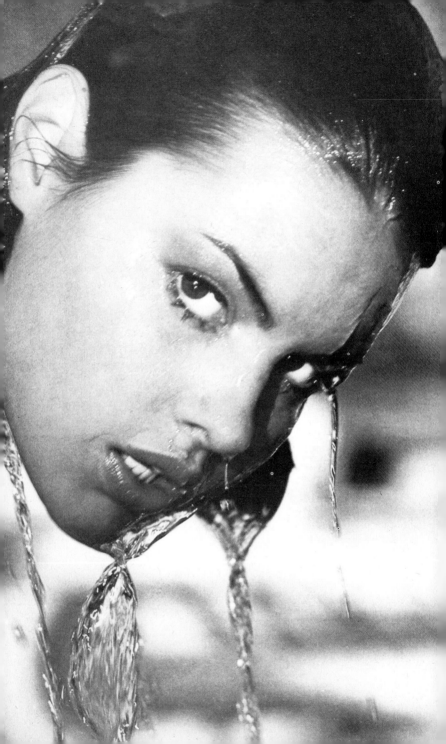

Skin Care:
How to Treat Each Type

All skin will look better if a regular routine is followed, and the earlier it is started, the longer skin will keep its elasticity and youth. Teenagers need to learn that regular cleansing and moisturizing is as important as cleaning their teeth – and the sooner they learn about their skin type and its problems, the fewer they will suffer as they grow older.

Whatever your age, once you've discovered your skin type and chosen the products you are going to use, you must work out a routine that you know can become a lifetime habit. Just like a diet, it's no good attempting something that doesn't fit into your life-style. Cleanse, tone and moisturize are the three basic steps to remember.

All skin needs cleansing – to get rid of surface dirt and stale make-up and to loosen clogged pores. You may be a soap and water addict, and there is nothing better than this, provided the soap is mild, designed for your skin type and thoroughly rinsed off afterwards. Or there are cleansers which also need to be rinsed off with water. Creams, greases and oils are good for dissolving make-up, particularly those specially formulated for removing eye make-up (where soap and water may irritate), but you then need a freshener as well to remove excess grease. These oil-based products are almost always used for removing heavy or theatrical make-up. Oils are often recommended for sensitive dry skins, but even these types can be cleansed with soap and water if the correct strength is used.

All skins need a freshener. After cleansing, a certain amount of debris and oil will inevitably remain and must be removed. Fresheners, toners and astringents are all of the same family, containing more or less alcohol. They are alcohol-free for dry and sensitive skins, contain a small amount for combination or balanced skins, and more for oily skins, with the addition of anti-septic ingredients for blemished skins. They all aim to stimulate circulation and restore the acid mantle which may have become unbalanced in the cleansing process.

All skins need moisturizing. Natural moisture evaporates and needs containing in even the oiliest skin. Moisturizers form a film over the skin's surface, holding in the natural moisture and providing a smooth base for make-up or a protective barrier between the skin and the environment. There are lightweight, medium and heavier types of moisturizer – the richer ones being needed as the skin grows older, or if they are going to be used without the added protection of foundation.

Specialized Care for Oily Skin
Oily skin with its tendency to shine and break out needs the most efficient deep cleansing. It's a good idea to use a cleanser formulated especially for this skin type, and since it may need cleansing midday as well as night and morning, choose one that's effective but not harsh. Follow with an astringent to remove any last traces of oil, but avoid the eye area. Oily skins need moisturizing too, to help the skin retain its natural moisture and stop it evaporating too fast. A lightweight moisturizer that leaves a matt surface on the skin is the one to look for, and if you find it too rich for daytime use, try using it only at night.

Even if oily skin persists as you get older, you will need eye and throat creams for those areas to combat wrinkles.

The use of a cleansing mask twice a week will help clear clogged pores, remove dead cells and refine the skin's texture.

Specialized Care for Blemished Skin

Basic care is the same as for oily skin, with the addition of medicated lotions to fight the bacteria that are causing problems. If the condition is severe, professional advice should be sought from a trained beautician, who may recommend medical help from your doctor or a dermatologist.

Specialized Care for Dry Skin

To keep dry skin at its delicate best, give it a good gentle cleansing night and morning. Night cleansing is very important since you have a day's accumulation of dirt and make-up to remove. A mild soap-and-water rinseable cleanser or cleansing cream is good for dry skin. Follow this with a light, non-alcoholic freshener – avoid anything called an astringent. A rich moisturizer should be used during the day, a nourishing cream at night, with specialized creams for eyes and throat.

A weekly exfoliating treatment will help to reduce flakiness, and a stimulating mask will encourage the glands to produce more natural lubricants.

Specialized Care for Sensitive Skin

Basic care is the same as for dry skin, with special attention to allergies. Look for sun-care and other products in hypoallergenic ranges. Most large cosmetic companies put their products through extensive allergy tests before putting them on the market, but those marked hypoallergenic are further tested for less common allergies.

Specialized Care for Combination Skin

Combination skin consists of dry and oily patches which need separate care. It is caused by the natural concentration of glands being heavier in some parts of the face than in others – normally in a T-shaped area across the forehead and down the nose. It is often too expensive to have different products for each area, so the answer is to use mild soap and water, or a cleanser that is not too abrasive for the dry areas but will clean the oily areas too. A mild toner, either non-alcoholic or with a small amount which can be diluted with water for the dry patches, is useful to remove excess grease and stimulate the circulation. Then, a medium-rich moisturizer is essential, concentrating on the dry parts, plus a special cream for eye area and neck. A clearing mask once a week down the centre panel will make all the difference to the balance of the skin.

Specialized Care for Balanced Skin
Basic care is the same as for dry skin, as even the best-behaved has a tendency to dry out as it grows older. To keep it at its best, a good cleanse, tone and moisturize routine is essential, and a weekly stimulating-mask treatment will encourage it to keep up the good work.

All skin types will benefit from an occasional visit to a beauty salon for a deep-cleanse treatment. The professional beautician will cleanse the skin, perhaps using the latest electronic equipment and paying attention to blackheads and whiteheads; stimulate the circulation with light massage using fingers or mechanical aids; and choose a good mask to help the particular condition of your skin. It is a good idea to make your appointment when you know you needn't wear make-up for a good twelve or, even better, twenty-four hours afterwards. This gives the skin time to breathe and benefit from the treatment it has received. Another good idea is to change the products you use occasionally. Just as your body benefits from a change of diet from time to time, so does your skin. However, ranges are formulated to work together, i.e. the ingredients of cleanser, moisturizer and toner that one company makes are designed to complement each other, so your skin is more likely to gain maximum benefit from them together than if you mix the different brands; also, they need to be used for several months or until they need replacing, if they are to do the job for which they were intended.

Steve Svensson

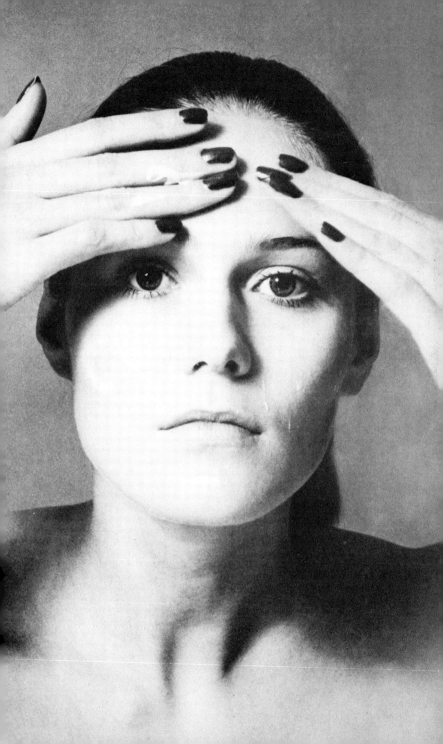

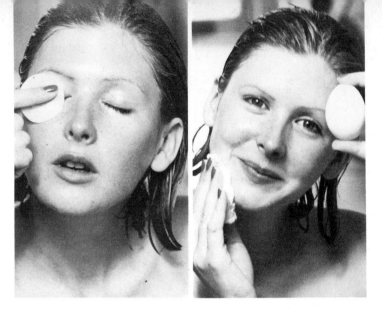

Cleansing pads *are good for removing mascara and stubborn eye make-up*

Toners and astringents *are after-cleansing agents for skin tightening and brightening*

Soap and water *give an unbeatable clean feeling; pure soaps won't dry or irritate the face*

Masks *strip off city grime, unclog pores and let the skin breathe*

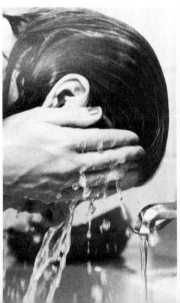
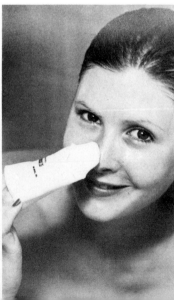

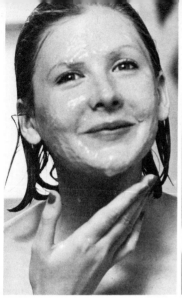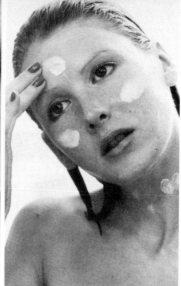

Gels *wake up sluggish skin and get it glowing*
Moisturizers *should be part of every skin's beauty routine morning and night*
Foams *are fluffy cleansers that whip on quickly*
All-in-ones *are multipurpose – a cleanser that's also a face-wash or shampoo; a moisturizer that works for face, legs and hands; a colour to highlight and blush*

Steve Svensson

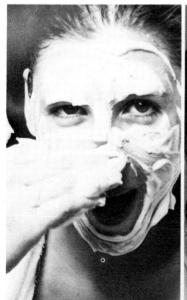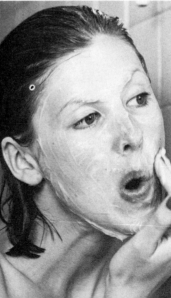

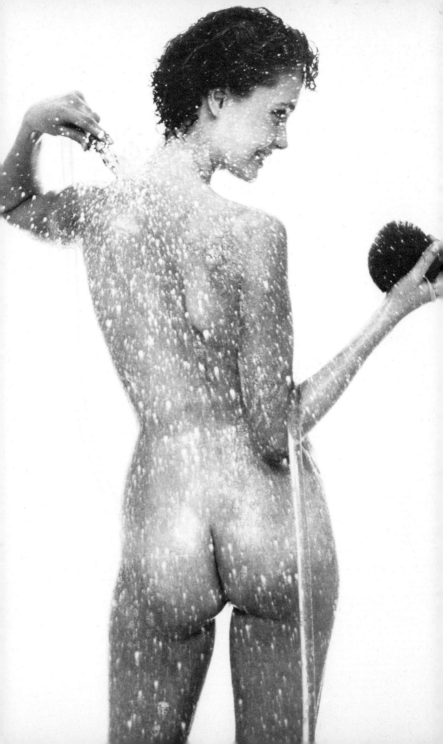

Cleansing the Body:
Baths and Showers

There is no question about it, all-over beauty begins in the bathroom. Cleansing the body is just as important as cleansing the face, and baths (or showers) are the only way to keep it clean and fresh. Most body odours, if allowed free access to fresh air, will evaporate quickly, and the smell, if any, will be quite pleasant. But, our civilization demands that our bodies are clothed 95 per cent of the time, and clothes (particularly those made of synthetic fibres) trap body moisture which quickly forms bacteria. It is the bacteria, not the sweat, that smell and become unpleasant. Deodorants are one way to attack the problem, but regular washing goes a long way towards solving it.

The bathroom itself should be a most relaxing and comfortable room – not something shoved into the only space available, with no heat, cold linoleum and draughty windows. In America many people have their make-up table and hair accessories in the bathroom too, thus making it a beauty room rather than merely functional. This sensible idea, along with proper lighting surrounding good mirrors, is gradually being adopted in Europe, and even existing cheerless bathrooms can be improved now there are wall-heaters, washable wall coverings and carpets, and now that draughts can be excluded. Mirrors are pretty (and an essential aid to beauty), certain plants thrive in the steamy atmosphere of a bathroom and well-placed lighting does much to ease pressure and tension. Take a new look at your bathroom and see what can be improved, then start discovering the pleasures of the bath.

Never try to get into a bath that is too hot, or stay in a hot bath too long. It is enervating and draws away too much of the body's natural moisture and oil, leaving you exhausted, your skin dry and often wrinkled.

A warm bath is best (not over 100°F or 38°C) as a general rule. A lukewarm bath is refreshing on very hot days (much more so than a cold dip, which has only a temporary effect) and a tepid one is a good pick-up at any time. Cold baths are traditionally bracing and cold water is easiest to brave under a shower – this is most stimulating, and if you can get really strong pressure from the water, it will not only improve circulation but exercise muscles too.

If your only object is to clean your body, then all you need is soap and water and something to dry it – sunshine or a towel. Possibly, if you are short of time, this is the sort of bath you need occasionally, but it takes no more time to add a moisturizing oil while it is running, and to use a fragrant soap. However, cleansing is not the only function of baths. Baths can relax the mind and muscles, soften and nourish the skin, stimulate the circulation, invigorate the mind and clear the head – which you choose usually depends on the time of day and the amount of time you can allow yourself, plus a thought for your general state of health.

First thing in the morning you need a good start to the day – it may be a *soothing transition* from sleep, in which case fragrant oils are a good idea, and an unhurried soak in warm water. Or, you may need a *brisk wake-up* and toner for relaxed muscles, so try a citrus or pine-scented essence in lukewarm water. Or, if your system needs a *real shock* to get it started, smooth over a body shampoo, rinse off under the shower with warm water, then turn the tap sharply to cold.

After a rough day, you need at least ten minutes for a *quiet bath* (remember to take the telephone off the hook, put on some gentle music and make sure you are not disturbed). This will revitalize you for the evening, and if you choose a hot bath, try and take a cool rinse afterwards for extra energy. A home-made infusion of herbs specially mixed for their soothing, calming, moisturizing properties is excellent at this time. Use dried herbs – grow your own and dry them, or buy them ready-dried. Then put your mixture in a muslin bag and tie it firmly to the hot tap so the water runs through it. Your *herbal bath* should include flowers as well as leaves (picked from roses, camomiles or lavender, elders or lemon-trees), pine-needles and any herbs you discover and like, such as fennel, thyme, rosemary, sage and peppermint. For instance, try a blackberry bath as a tonic for your skin ... make a strong infusion and use it for two or three nights running. A pine bath to refresh ... boil pine-needles for half an hour and allow them to steep overnight; strain and use a cupful in each bath. A lemon bath to invigorate ... add slices to a lemon-scented bath oil and use slices to rub over your skin. An elder bath for soothing ... in infusion form. A lavender bath for pleasure ... dried lavender flowers mixed with a little dried mint and rosemary. Alternatively, choose one of the ready-mixed herbal concoctions available or the delicious products which include herbs in the ingredients. Last thing before bed, a *lazy warm bath* encourages sleep – it should be redolent of sweet-smelling flowers, with moisturizing foam or milk. Pat yourself dry afterwards – don't rub vigorously and don't take your bath too soon after a meal. There are variations to try at any time:

The country bath. Everyone knows what a day in the country does for morale and beauty. A country-smelling bath allows you to dream yourself into the same state. Without taking a step you can conjure up fields of flowers, old-fashioned herb gardens, a glade of bluebells or hedgerow of honeysuckle, wild roses and moss. Try gels that blend extracts of marigold and pine-needles, soften the water and cleanse the body ... essences that soften and scent the water ... oils that soften, cleanse and nourish the skin.

A flowery bath. There's nothing more delightful than to receive a beautiful bouquet of flowers. Almost as good, but better for your skin, is a fragrantly flowery bath. Choose a milk bath with the bouquet of honeysuckle, rose and spices – and use talcum powder, body cream and deodorant in matching fragrance to help the scent linger ... a foam bath or oil to soften or to colour your bath a delicious sea-blue or green.

A sea-water bath, if you long for that breezy tang of a holiday. There are lots of bath additives using sea algae, which contain all the minerals of sea water that help draw toxic substances from the body and ease rheumatic complaints, aching joints and muscles.

As with everything else, you need the right equipment to get the most out of your bath: a rough-textured loofah, perfect for removing dead skin and leaving the body tingling; a sponge for soaping your skin (when it becomes clogged with soap, steep overnight in vinegar to freshen it); nail-brush and body brush – choose them with stiff, natural bristles; pumice-stone for rubbing away rough skin on heels, soles of the feet and elbows; flannel or bath mitt made of cotton towelling for rubbing on soap (make sure you launder them frequently or they'll harden with the soap residue).

After your bath your skin is at its most receptive – this is the moment, when it is completely dry, to use a deodorant, lots of moisturizing body lotion, a splash of cologne and talcum powder; if your finger- or toenails need cutting, they are soft and pliant after a bath, and it is a good moment to massage cuticles with a nourishing cream.

Barry Lategan

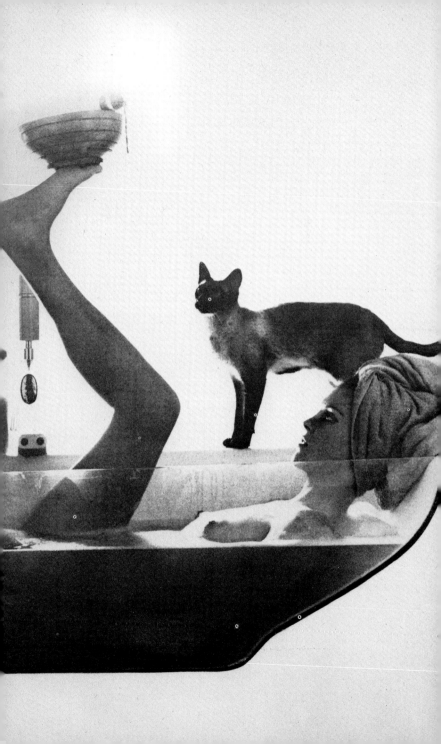

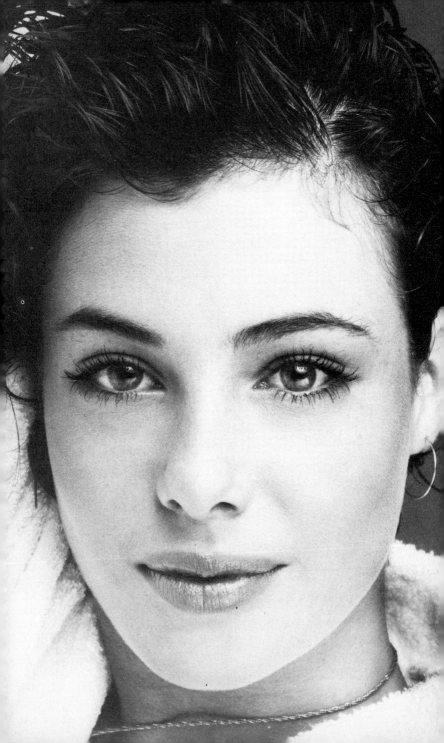

Beauty Products:
What Does What Do to Your Face?

Basic beauty kit for taking proper care of the skin on your face should include cleanser, eye make-up remover, toner, moisturizer, plus (depending on your age and individual needs) night cream, eye cream, throat cream and various masks.

Cleansers. There are foam cleansers, gel cleansers, cream cleansers, milky cleansers, cleansing oils and, of course, the original soap and water routine. (The modern cleansing bar is totally non-alkaline and contains no soap of any kind. It can be used in any kind of water, hard or soft. It contains an emulsifying agent similar to that used in a cleansing cream, plus solidifying agents that turn the cream into a bar.) Which you use is a matter of personal preference, but the point of cleansing your skin is to clean it. New-born babies are bathed and cleaned with oils; children and teenagers, even before starting to use make-up, should learn to clean their face, not just to remove visible food or dirt but all over, to clear it of grime accumulated during the day which, if allowed to become ingrained, will cause spots and blackheads. Later it becomes obvious that stale make-up needs removing thoroughly and the skin needs frequent cleansing.

Special eye make-up removers. These become necessary as more and more people want water- or smudge-proof make-up. This make-up clings to the face and so becomes more difficult to remove, and ordinary cleansers, particularly soap and water, have a tendency to irritate the eyes. There are creams, oils and liquids to choose from – also boxes of pads saturated with a cleanser which are neat and easy to use.

Toners. Either an alcohol-free freshener, a mild toner or an astringent is necessary to remove any traces of cleanser, to close the pores and generally brighten up the skin's texture before the application of moisturizer.

Moisturizers. These help to replace the natural moisture lost through evaporation and act as a barrier protecting the skin from air pollution or as a preparatory base for foundation, making it easier to blend in and look natural.

Night creams. These are a richer form of moisturizer containing extra lubricants to help combat wrinkles and ageing. Young people and sufferers from oily skin often find a day-time moisturizer sufficient for night-time use.

Eye creams and throat creams are nourishing creams specially formulated to feed the skin in those areas. They are usually used at night, although the newer formulations are less and less greasy and are often recommended for day-time use too.

Masks can cleanse, revitalize, condition, stimulate or exfoliate. They are applied all over the face, avoiding the eye area and mouth, left to dry for a certain time and then either rinsed or peeled off. They are always included in a professional facial when the type will be decided for you, but for home use be sure you buy the variety you want.

Cleansing masks have a deep-down action, helping to free clogged pores, loosen blackheads, remove surface dirt and clear dead cells.

Revitalizing masks often provide the quick pick-up your face needs before going out for the evening; they can be applied before a bath and will have done their job by the time you are out and dry – in about 10–15 minutes.

Conditioning masks do just that. They give your face an occasional deep treat and are particularly good if you don't use a night cream, as they provide the extra nourishment your skin needs.

Stimulating masks purify the skin and activate circulation, pumping more oxygen to the surface and leaving the blood-vessels

Mike Reinhardt (opposite), *Albert Watson* (overleaf)

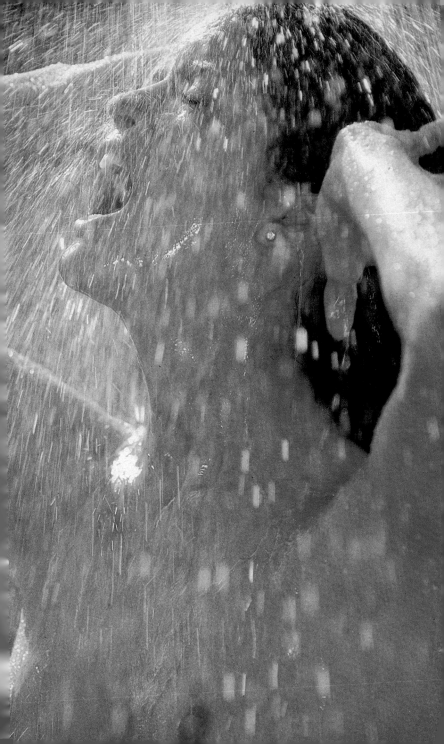

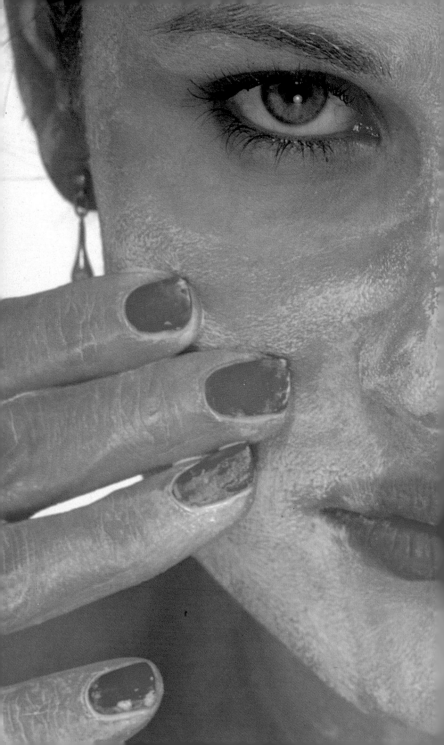

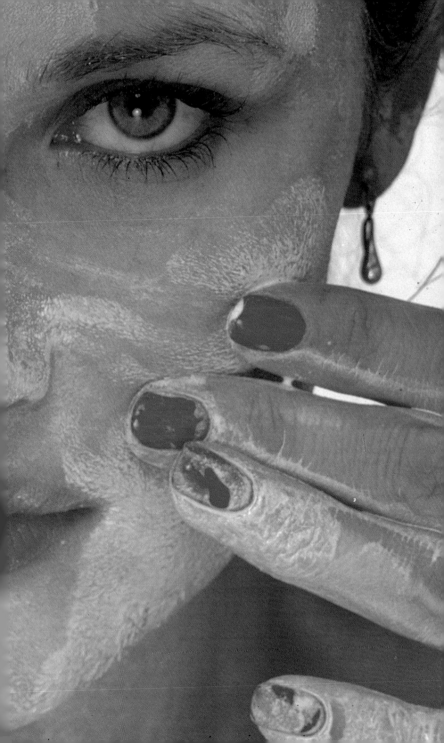

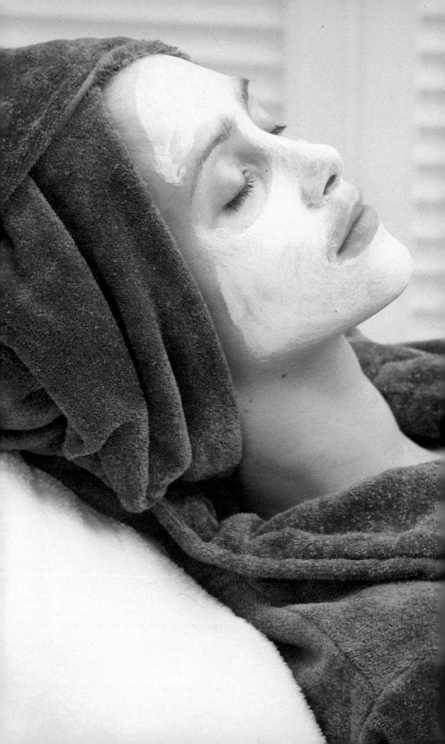

enlarged so that the skin will look pink when it's removed. This increased circulation will improve the skin's colour and texture.

Exfoliating masks are designed especially for the removal of dead cells from the surface of the skin and are really a gentle form of peeling (only practised to get rid of lines, soften scars and remove blemishes, and only done by qualified specialists). The dead cells are what often give the skin a grey look or blotchy tone, and the use of an exfoliating mask will brighten the appearance and smooth the texture.

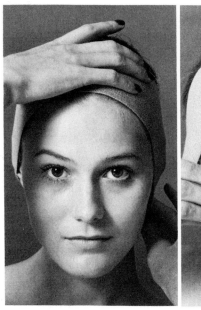 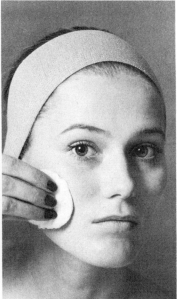

Step-by-Step Facial

1. Put a headband or tie a scarf around your hairline to keep hair out of face and lotions out of hair. 2. Apply a gentle cleanser with a cotton-wool pad. To do this the professional way, use motions that 'cut across'

John Swannell (opposite)
William Connors (above)

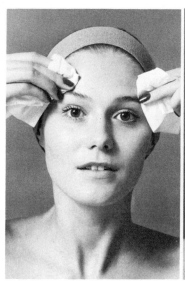
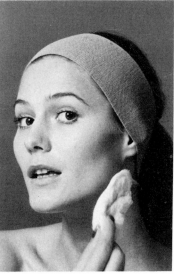

skin lines and wrinkles. Use up and down strokes on forehead, horizontal movements above lips and on chin, and for the eye area, a motion that starts at cheek, comes towards nose and up across brows. These movements help to discourage more wrinkles and should be used both when applying and when removing skin-care products. **3.** *Tissue off the cleanser, making sure to use the motions described.* **4.** *Apply a toner to remove last traces of cleanser and tighten pores slightly. You are now ready for a mask.* **5.** *(opposite) Put on a light moisturizer, dotting it on forehead, cheeks and chin, then blending it in with fingertips. Again use the motions described.* **6.** *Rinse skin with clear luke-warm water, then apply mask. Leave on for prescribed time and relax.* **7.** *To make the most of your rest, apply cotton-wool pads soaked in skin tonic to your eyes for a soothing, cool feeling.* **8.** *Remove mask and blot – do not rub face with a towel. Finish off with a thin film of moisturizer.*

34

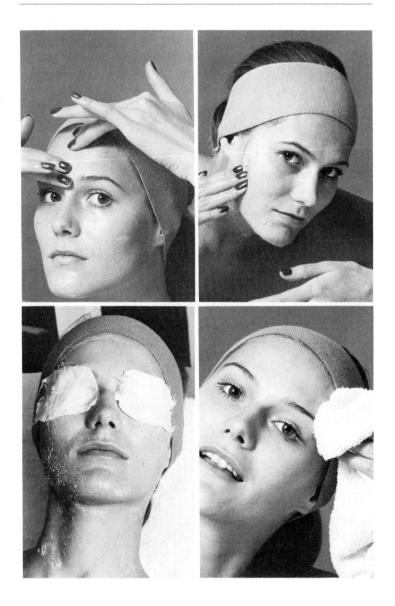

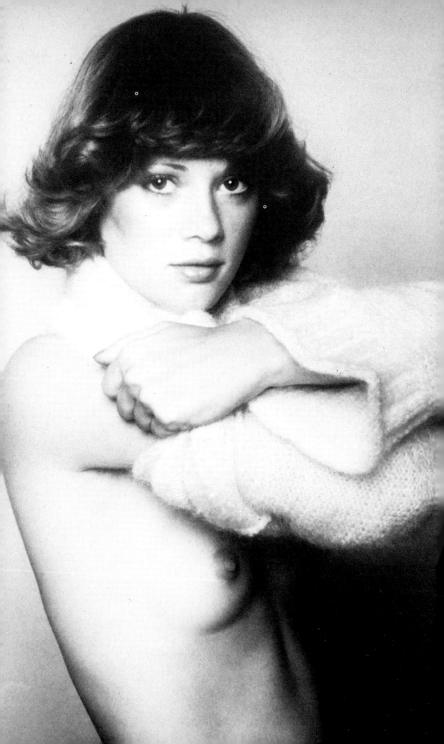

Age:
What Happens When?

Most of us are lucky and were born whole. We contain all the proper organs (intestines, glands, veins, blood and so on), we have features and limbs and hair where they should be and our skin is unblemished. In fact we have everything intended for the perfect human being – and it's all in good working order. But, as we grow older, the body becomes used and abused, and changes take place. Skin, in particular, goes through phases and is susceptible to various problems at these times. Even babies may suffer early from rashes, allergies and problems related to their skin type which continue through childhood.

Teens

Puberty causes a tremendous upheaval in the body, with hormonal activity affecting every gland and consequently the skin. Skin, which until now may have behaved beautifully, suddenly starts playing up and erupting into *acne*. This is the result of hormones stimulating the oil glands into over-production of oil, which gets clogged in the pores. This is so prevalent among adolescents – girls and boys – that it is often dismissed as something they must just endure until it goes away. But, treatment is available, and if the course is followed properly, the skin condition will certainly improve and, depending on its severity, may disappear. Another problem connected with this hormonal activity is that the *hair* follicles all over the body are stimulated into growth and it sometimes appears in unwanted places – above the upper lip and on the sides of the face, for instance. However, once the body has settled into its new pattern, this facial hair often falls out and doesn't return; if it is dark and very obvious it can be lightened with a special facial hair bleach, but more serious forms of removal should be left for several years.

Enlarged pores, sometimes a symptom of oily skin, sometimes resulting from acne, but caused by excess oil clogging and then stretching the pores, are also a sign of adolescence. They don't disappear, so scrupulous cleansing to prevent their arrival is the answer. Another condition – seen by some as a problem, by others as an attractive asset – is freckles. These often go hand in hand with the pale translucent skin possessed by natural red-heads and are actually cells containing extra quantities of melanin (a dark pigment stimulated by sunlight into turning brown) grouped together in the skin. They will increase in the sunshine, but often fade in the winter months and can only temporarily be removed. However, a good sun block (see p. 65) will help to curtail their numbers.

Twenties
This is when your skin should look its best – it has been through the upheaval of adolescence and is not yet on the road to decline, although it will show signs of ageing in the late twenties if care is not taken. In fact most problems that appear now are caused by lack of care in the teens. Neglect during those years, and sometimes the use of cosmetics designed for a more mature skin (borrowed from mother perhaps, or lent with the best intentions) can result in *acne* appearing now. Or it can be the result of going on the Pill.

If *freckles* or *brown spots* appear at this stage and seem to be the variety that don't fade in winter, they aren't natural and are probably caused by over-exposure to the sun, which will also hasten the ageing process later on. These blemishes are removable by a dermatologist, but after treatment great care should be taken not to expose the skin to the sun.

Skin allergies usually become apparent in the twenties – when

38

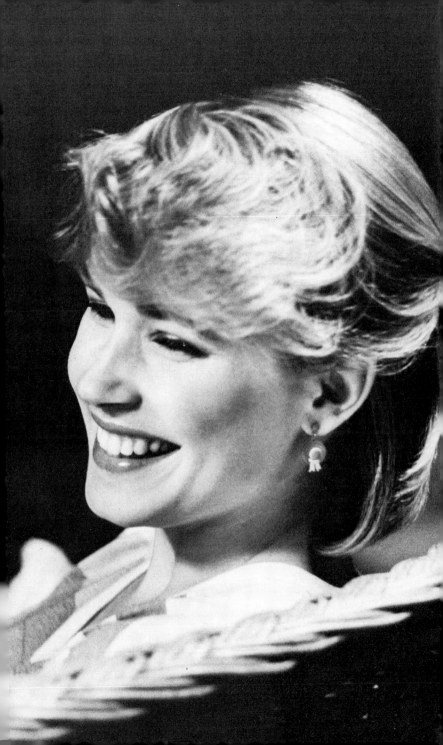

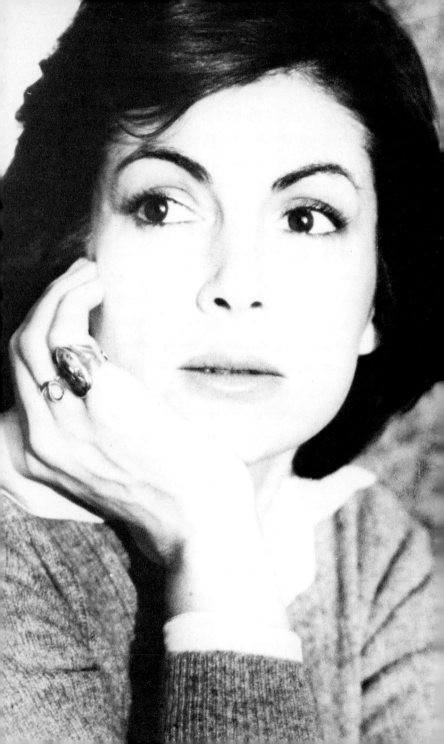

women have started working in offices or factories or running their own homes and thus handle industrial equipment and office machinery or have contact with detergents, insecticides and so on. They often continue to use many different cosmetics and fragrances; they may travel more, experimenting with foreign foods. Any of these may cause an allergic reaction. The way to treat an allergy is to isolate it, then protect yourself as much as possible. This may involve a series of allergy tests to discover the cause.

Thirties

This is the time to guard against skin drying out and causing premature ageing. Change your skin-care routine to one for-mulated for more mature skins and watch out for a variety of acne called *dry skin acne*. This is thought to be caused by a special kind of oil, containing quantities of fatty acids, irritating the pores. Dry skin acne takes the form of blackheads and whiteheads, mostly on the chin and jaw-line. Women who have had dry skin all their lives will probably start noticing lines – fine ones, but lines all the same – and *bags* may appear under the eyes, removable only by cosmetic surgery, although, if caused by fluid from allergy or sinus problems, antihistamines can sometimes prevent the formation of these pouches.

Broken blood vessels, due to skin damage from pregnancy, excess alcohol, high blood pressure or a blow to the skin, may begin to show on the cheeks and around the nose as small red lines. These can usually be treated by a doctor.

Forties

The skin is beginning to lose its tone and strength – it finds it difficult to support the pores, and they start becoming more visible and may become *enlarged*. Masks and astringents will help temporarily. Another variety of acne – *acne rosacea* – often appears during the forties. Its exact cause is not known, although stress, alcohol, spicy foods and extremes of hot and cold are known to aggravate the condition. It has a flushed appearance with blackheads and small pustules and can be treated by a dermatologist. *Psoriasis* also, although it can occur at any age, is most likely to appear now, its round red patches flecked with silvery scales showing first on elbows and knees. It is very difficult to cure.

Fifties and Onwards

The skin must begin to show its age however well it's been looked-after. It is no longer receiving sufficient support and elasticity from the protein fibres, and the fatty deposits beneath the skin are disappearing, leaving it loose and flabby. Lines deepen into *wrinkles*, the skin dries and the *drying skin* itself becomes a problem, sometimes with painful side-effects like itching, a slowness to heal and a tendency to become infected. Little clusters of *red lines* called *spider angiomata* may appear, as may *brown spots*. Deterioration in skin colour is often due to poor circulation and can be improved by massage and exercise. Most serious of all, this is the time when *skin cancer* usually appears. Of the four basic types, *solar keratoses*, which manifests itself in rough red patches, is the mildest. It is most commonly found in people who have sunbathed too much and for too long, people involved in outdoor sports or who lead outdoor lives. It can be treated but if left too long can develop into the more serious *squamous cell carcinoma*, a thicker, rougher growth. Both these types usually show first on the face – which is also usually the first area to be affected by a persistent sore that doesn't heal called *basal cell carcinoma*. All three types are treatable, but the last two may leave some scarring. The last type, and fortunately the least common, as it is by far the most serious, is *malignant melanoma*. The first sign is a deeply pigmented area on the skin coloured brown, black or even dark blue, which acts as a warning that there is a growth. A lump which changes colour or size when exposed to the sun may also indicate this type of cancer and should be checked immediately. The treatment is to remove the growth and a large area of the skin which surrounds it.

Arthur Elgort

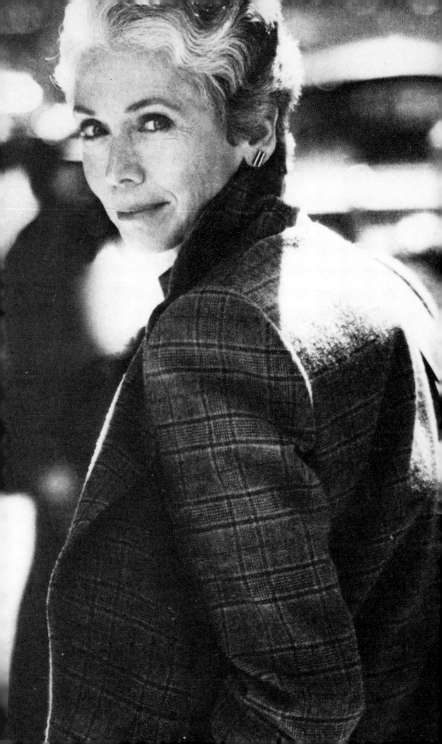

An A–Z of Common Skin Problems

Acne

Treatment for acne has developed tremendously in recent years. The condition is caused by over-activity of the sebaceous glands, which causes too much oil to flow, thus clogging and irritating the pores. Its occurrence is easily understandable during the hormonal changes undergone in adolescence; less easy to understand are the types of acne that flare up later. These vary with the age at which they appear. It is now thought that an exaggerated emphasis has been put on the connection between foods, such as chocolate, and acne and that the condition is not usually caused by dirt.

Teenage acne is synonymous with adolescence and causes much distress. Modern treatment discourages abrasive and over-zealous cleaning as this is thought to over-stimulate the oil glands into renewed activity. Gentle washing in conjunction with a special lotion has a better long-term effect. Low doses of the antibiotic oxytetracycline are frequently prescribed by doctors and dermatologists and are effective in alleviating severe acne. So too is a treatment involving retinoic acid. This works by loosening and softening the hardened keratin which is plugging the pores and causing the acne. Teenage acne should clear by the age of twenty-one, but if it hasn't it's likely to go on well into the thirties.

Acne which appears during the twenties is sometimes caused by birth-control pills, neglect of the skin during the teenage years or by the use of rich cosmetics designed for a more mature skin and inadequate cleansing.

Stress acne is likely to occur in the thirties; it appears suddenly in the form of large painful cysts with no accompanying blackheads, pustules or oily skin. Women under stress can, overnight, find their normally clear skin in trouble. One treatment is to inject the cyst with cortisone.

Dry skin acne is also common at this age – contradicting the idea that acne and oily skin are linked. This kind of acne is caused by a specific kind of oil, thought to contain large amounts of fatty acids, which irritates the pores until they erupt, usually into blackheads and whiteheads around the chin and jaw-line. This is normally treated with a low dose of tetracycline.

Acne rosacea is most likely to attack in the forties – arriving with a rosy flush and quickly followed by blackheads and small pustules. Its exact cause isn't known, but alcohol, spicy foods, stress and tension, extreme heat or intense cold are thought to aggravate the condition. Low doses of tetracycline will suppress the problem and a sulphur lotion is often helpful.

Extreme symptoms – excessively oily skin, facial hair, large quantities of cysts, for instance – indicate a real hormonal disorder, and dermatologists will often refer these cases to specialists to determine the cause before treating the problem further.

Allergies

One widespread cause of skin distress is allergic reaction. If you break out in spots or rashes, the cause may be something you have eaten or just touched; this is known as contact allergy. *Where* the outbreak occurs is often a clue to the problem – with the common nickel allergy, for instance, a reaction may appear just where a belt buckle or jeans fastener touched the skin. Skin allergies often become apparent in the twenties – after a few years in an office, factory or running a home and being in contact with office equipment, industrial machinery or everyday products like detergents. And by this time some women have developed an allergy to certain cosmetics – nail-polish is a well-known example,

45

showing not around the fingers, but where they touch the face (around the eyes, lips, etc.). As a rule modern cosmetics are very safe to use, being stringently tested before they are put on the market and using formulae which avoid any known irritants. To treat an allergy, the cause must be identified, and if it's not quickly obvious, this may entail a series of tests prescribed by a dermatologist, usually done in groups of patches on the back.

Athlete's Foot
This is a kind of ringworm that thrives in warm damp areas – most commonly found between toes and on the soles of the feet, occasionally between fingers. It is an infection picked up from going barefoot in communal areas, when enough care hasn't been taken to dry the feet after being immersed in water, or when they have sweated into socks that are left unchanged. The skin looks white and opaque, can itch and forms thick blisters which peel.

Bags
Under-eye bags are often hereditary, but during the thirties they can appear as a result of severe allergy or sinus problems where fluid is emptied into the area; this stretches the delicate skin, which loses its ability to spring back and so sags. The only real treatment for these pouches is cosmetic surgery.

Blackheads
Blackheads are not coloured by dirt but by melanin, the substance that makes skin and hair the colour they are. The darker your skin, the blacker they will be (very fair people are less prone to them as their skins are usually drier as well). They should not be prodded or poked as this is likely to cause enlargement and infection. Gentle, thorough cleansing softens the plug, bringing it to the surface and making it easy to rinse away; persistent blackheads should be treated by a trained beautician.

Blushing

This is a common physical sign of what's going on emotionally in the head – normally embarrassment, shame or anger. Some people only suffer on the face; with others the face remains pale while the chest starts to go red and the blush creeps up the neck. It is frustrating, and nothing has yet been discovered to control it – *you* certainly can't.

Blotchy Skin

If this only appears occasionally on the face, neck or chest it is probably an emotional blush, but if it is more widespread and permanent it is probably due to bad circulation. Massage and exercise will probably help.

Brown Spots

Brown spots appear on sun-abused skin in early life – the twenties – and are a normal part of skin ageing as you grow older. There are creams which can fade them and they can be removed without scarring by a dermatologist.

Cellulite

This is sometimes called *peau d'orange* because the skin over the affected area has the crinkly appearance of orange peel. The condition is caused by deposits of stubborn fat and excess water-retention accumulating beneath the skin, most likely on thighs, hips, buttocks and the upper arms. It affects thin as well as fat people and is very difficult to dislodge permanently. Massage alone is seldom very helpful as it often just moves the problem from one area to another. Breaking up and dissolving the deposits by a combination of exercise, diet and specialized salon treatment is the only effective way to reduce it, while healthy eating and proper exercise from an early age are the best ways to avoid it. Keeping a check on fluid-retention by eating foods that contain potassium (which helps excrete excess salt) and drinking lots of good mineral water is also a good idea.

Corns
There are hard corns and soft corns – hard ones usually appear on joints, soft ones between toes – which grow on feet as a warning against ill-fitting shoes. Pressure causes a hardening of the skin which, if left unrelieved (special felt circles are widely available for this), will form a horny corn with the apex pointing inwards. Further pressure put on this apex causes intense pain. Corns should be treated by a chiropodist – amateur cutting and scraping can result in infection.

Cysts
These appear as solid little lumps either under the skin, usually the result of blocked sweat-glands, or in the ovaries where, if not detected and removed, they can grow to enormous sizes. There is a variety called a ganglion which usually appears near joints, e.g. on the hands near the wrists. These are filled with a clear jelly-like substance and can easily be removed surgically.

Dermatitis or Eczema
This is an inflammation of the skin that can appear anywhere on the body; it is red and often produces a mass of small blister-like bumps or dry scaly skin. There are many variations. The usual cause is an external irritant, i.e. an allergy to something in the sufferer's daily life, but nerves and emotions are also closely connected.

Enlarged Pores
These are caused by a permanent stretching of pores clogged by excess oil and often result from acne – even the mildest attack. Like anything else that is stretched beyond its capacity to spring back, once a pore becomes enlarged it is impossible to reduce it.

Prevention by careful cleansing and immediate attention to any problem is essential.

Facial Hair
This is often a teenage problem resulting from the hormonal changes occurring in the body and is most often seen around the upper lip and along the sides of the face. Once the hormones have settled down, this hair often falls out, never to return, but if it is dark and unsightly it can safely be lightened with a specifically formulated bleach. More drastic forms of removal such as electrolysis or waxing should be left until the problem appears to have become permanent at the end of adolescence.

Flabby Skin
This can appear in the young as a result of lack of exercise and poor diet and can be tightened up with a course of regular exercises and massage if these steps are taken soon enough. Flabby skin is also often the result of sudden weight-loss through illness or a too drastic diet and a return to fitness will depend on age and the amount of elasticity remaining in the skin.

Freckles
Certain people – often red-heads – are born with skin prone to freckles, which are groups of cells in the skin containing above-normal amounts of the dark pigment called melanin. They will fade in the winter, increase in the summer, can be reduced with a mild chemical peeling, but will return on re-exposure to sunlight. They are often very attractive, but if the possessor wants to keep them to a minimum, the use of a sun block (see p. 65) is essential in spring and summer. Freckles that appear later in life are called Brown Spots (see p. 47).

Frostbite
This is caused by exposure to intense cold and the stoppage of the

blood flow in vessels close to the skin's surface. The affected area – most often nose, fingers, toes or ears – becomes white, hard and numb and, if not treated fast, will cause permanent damage to the skin. The best treatment is to restore circulation with very gentle warmth such as bathing in cool water, although the area will become painfully inflamed and may produce rupturing blisters. Minor frostbite can be prevented by wearing enough suitable warm loose-fitting clothes to keep circulation going and, if skiing, for instance, in very cold conditions, frequently checking any exposed areas on yourself or your companions.

Lines
These are usually noticed around the eye area in the thirties and can come from allergies or sinus problems, particularly in conjunction with under-eye bags, or from worry or shock. Keeping the area well-moisturized with an eye cream is preventative or can delay their premature deepening. Later, around the fifties, when lines are deepening around the nose and mouth and everything seems to be sagging from a lessening of elasticity, a face-lift is the only solution.

Moles
Moles are flat or slightly raised patches of dark pigmentation which can be unsightly if too bumpy or if they sprout a few hairs. The hairs shouldn't be pulled out nor should any attempt be made at home removal of the mole – they are easy to remove safely if professionally done. Most moles are harmless, but a flat mole that changes colour or size or bleeds should be medically checked immediately.

Perspiration
The body's natural heat-controlling, air-conditioning system, this is the liquid produced by the sweat-glands – regularly appearing in armpits and groin, and after exercise or specific stimulation of the

body temperature (from a sauna, for instance) occurring all over the body. The liquid is odourless but, if constricted by clothing or trapped by a fold of skin or joint, will quickly form bacteria; it is this that smells. When fresh, this smell is considered quite attractive by some, but, if allowed to become stale or dry into clothes that are worn again before being washed or cleaned, it is always unpleasant. Fat people perspire more than thin and a diet will obviously help; others come out in a 'cold sweat' from fear or emotional stress, often around the hairline and across the forehead. Excessive non-induced sweating needs medical treatment. There are excellent antiperspirants and deodorant-antiperspirants on the market, but as perspiring is a very important part of the body's natural cooling-system, you should use the mildest antiperspirant you can. Everyone differs in how much they sweat and, of course, it is a real problem for some: those who sweat excessively need the strongest possible deterrent, but most people just need a little help to control the flow and prevent a bad smell.

Red Lines
These usually appear around the nose and cheeks in the thirties and are broken surface blood-vessels caused by skin damage (windburn, frostbite), pregnancy, alcohol or high blood pressure. They can often be treated by a doctor or trained beautician inexpensively and relatively painlessly, using an electric needle and special chemical fluid to drain the blood-vessel. A serious condition, in the legs for instance, may need several sessions and take time. Later, a variety called spider angiomata, which radiate from a central red point, may appear but can be removed by cauterization.

Scars
Whenever the skin is damaged – cut, burned or stretched – it will leave a scar. Surface scars will disappear without trace (particularly in the young); deeper wounds, where the tissue is destroyed,

will leave permanent marks. Stretch marks and minor scars are sometimes helped by a vitamin E oil or special cream. Severe disfiguring ones will need chemical peeling or skin-grafting, and medical advice must be sought.

Skin Cancer

This is most commonly found in women who have spent a lifetime sunbathing without due protection for their skin. *Solar keratoses* are rough, red patches which can be surgically removed safely and will heal leaving no scar. If left untreated these pre-cancerous lesions will develop into the far more serious *squamous cell carcinoma*, which is a thickened, roughened version of the above and mostly appears on the face.

Basal cell carcinoma also appears predominantly on the face as a persistent small sore. Both these conditions can be treated by surgery or chemotherapy, but some scarring may ensue.

The most severe and fortunately rarest form of skin cancer is called *malignant melanoma* and is indicated by deeply pigmented patches, coloured brown, black or sometimes dark blue, or by a lump which suddenly changes colour when exposed to the sun. Any patch should be checked by a doctor as speedily as possible since treatment involves removal of the affected area plus a certain amount of surrounding skin, depending on the state of the growth.

Skin Discolouration

A sallow skin tone may be improved by increasing the blood circulation; likewise a pale tone. Anything that increases the flow of blood and brings more to the surface will improve the effect and give the skin a pinker tint. Regular exercises, a good brisk walk or body massage all help. A ruddy complexion is difficult to reduce – although alcohol, coffee and spicy foods should be avoided – and as far as the face is concerned, there are coloured prefoundation creams designed to help.

Sunburn

Sunburn often shows the morning after a day spent in the sun, or in the evening when the first sign is a stinging as you get into a bath. It is a painful reddening of the skin (sometimes so sensitive that even a loose cotton shirt or sheet will hurt), followed by peeling.

Very fair skins are exceptionally sensitive to the sun, but anyone – even black skins that have been away from the sun for any length of time – can on occasion suffer from sunburn and heatstroke. Very fair skins should use a sun block, wear wide-brimmed hats and cover as much of the body as possible, but everyone who values the beauty of their skin should take sunbathing gently and always wear creams that will filter out the damaging ultra-violet rays. You can still go beautifully brown: it will just take a little longer.

Unwanted Hair

Hair growing on parts of the body – face, bikini-line, underarms and legs are common – where it isn't wanted can be disguised by bleaching, which is quite satisfactory if the original growth is reasonably fair; removed temporarily with suitable depilatory creams or stripped off with wax; or removed permanently by electrolysis, which is expensive and time-consuming but worth it for a small area or if the hair is causing exceptional distress. (See also p. 57ff.)

Veruccas

Infectious inward-growing warts on the feet, usually picked up by children or young adults who frequent communal changing-rooms in schools, sports centres, swimming-pools, etc. and walk around barefoot – one verucca will soon multiply into many more – they are painful and need attention from a chiropodist, who will treat them with an acid product, electronically or, as a last resort if the verucca grows very deep, surgically.

53

Warts
Small hard growths appearing often on hands or face, usually on children or teenagers and mostly caused by a virus, they often just disappear, if left untreated, but if too numerous or large to leave, they can be treated with special solutions, scraped, burned or cut off. The large, soft, moist variety that occasionally appears in the genital area should be treated by a doctor.

Whiteheads
First cousin to the blackhead, they are tiny, hard, white lumps just under the skin that cannot find an exit unless the pore is opened. They should not be tampered with at home, but a trained beautician will make an opening, remove the offending waxy mass and leave not a trace.

Windburn
Red, dry patches, usually on cheeks or exposed areas, appear as a result of exposure without protection to strong winds combined with glaring light. Sportspersons, such as all-weather skiers who venture out in blizzards, dinghy and ocean-racing sailors, cross-country riders and all athletes, need to take precautions to protect their skin from windburn.

Zymotic Disease
This is a now disused and archaic description (coined by 19th-century Dr William Parr before the discovery and identification of viruses) for epidemic, endemic and contagious diseases such as smallpox that assumed the similarity of fermentation (zymosis) and infection.

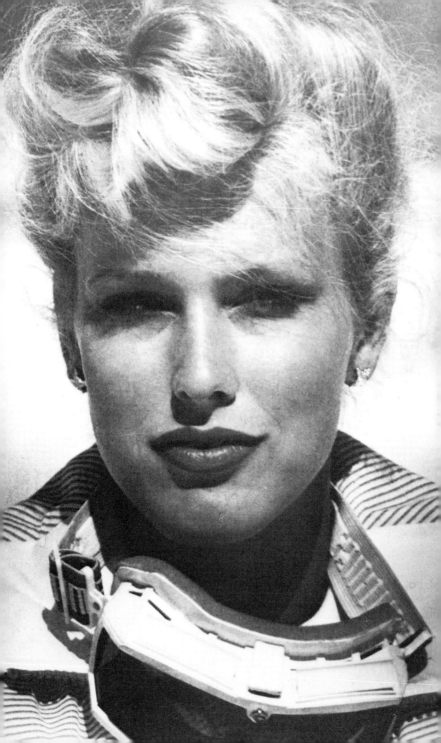

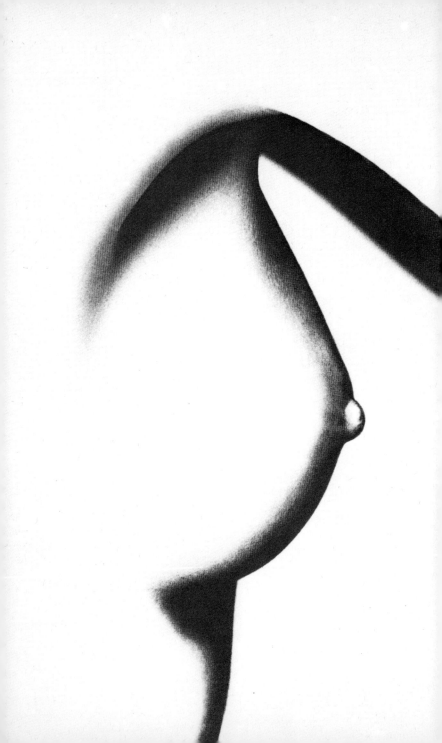

Unwanted Hair:
What to Do about It

While hair on the head is something to be admired, any profusion elsewhere on the body is in most cultures considered unattractive and something to be got rid of. Body hair is quite normal and can range from one persistent coarse hair on the chin, through a dark shadow on the upper lip, or eyebrows that meet across the bridge of the nose, to hair that grows around the nipples, under the arms, on arms, legs, fingers, toes, tummy and around the bikini-line.

There are various methods of removal to choose from.

Plucking
The easiest and most convenient way of removing stray hairs on face and breasts and it has no adverse effects, although, of course, the hair will reappear, and some people find it a slightly uncomfortable process. It is a good idea, before tweezing, to wipe the area with cotton-wool soaked in an astringent or a mild antiseptic; this will remove any oil and help you grip the smallest hair. Also, make sure you keep your tweezers scrupulously clean – wipe them also with the cotton-wool before using. Never try to remove hair that is sprouting from a mole or wart; this should be checked professionally.

Bleaching
This doesn't remove any hair but is an excellent method of disguising hair on face, arms, legs, and inner, upper thighs (the

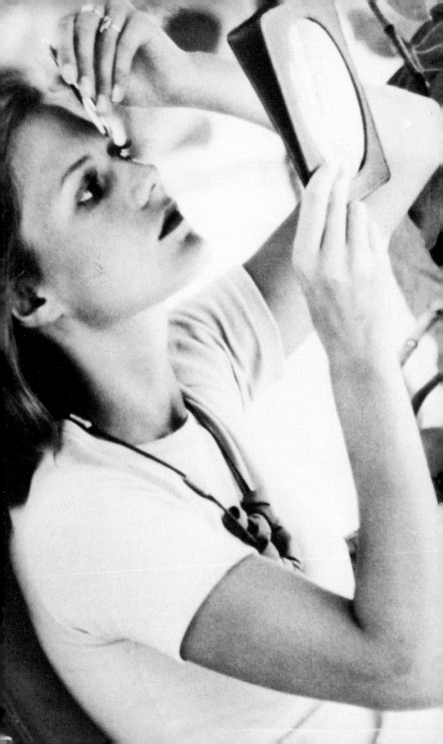

bikini area). There are good commercial products on the market, or you can make your own by mixing 30 per cent peroxide with a little ammonia and water (if you have even slightly sensitive skin, try a patch test a day in advance). Darker hair sometimes needs two applications.

Shaving

A simple and efficient way of removing underarm and leg hair, this shouldn't be used elsewhere, except where pubic hair is extending on to the upper thighs. The new hair does not grow faster or in more profusion or more coarsely, but, because it reappears with a blunt end from having been sliced off with the razor, it feels more bristly. In order to avoid cutting the skin, don't shave dry – lather the area with soap and water, use a new sharp blade and rinse and dry the skin carefully afterwards. Legs can be kept smooth with regular use of a pumice-stone – lather well, then rub the stone all over in circular movements.

Waxing

An ancient method of temporary hair removal, it is suitable for most parts of the body. (The wax is heated to a thin consistency, applied in strips, allowed to cool and then quickly ripped off, bringing the hairs with it.) It can be painful, particularly if you tend to retain water (just before getting a period, for instance), but it pulls the hair from beneath the skin's surface (although it doesn't destroy the roots) so re-growth takes longer and appears soft and smooth. Many people find that in time the re-growth is weakened and the amount of visible hair reduced. Ingrowing hairs are sometimes a problem, in which case bleaching is probably a more satisfactory method. Waxing is most efficiently done in professional salons, but wax can be bought and the process done at home; although time-consuming, it is quite satisfactory, particularly if you have a friend to help reach awkward areas.

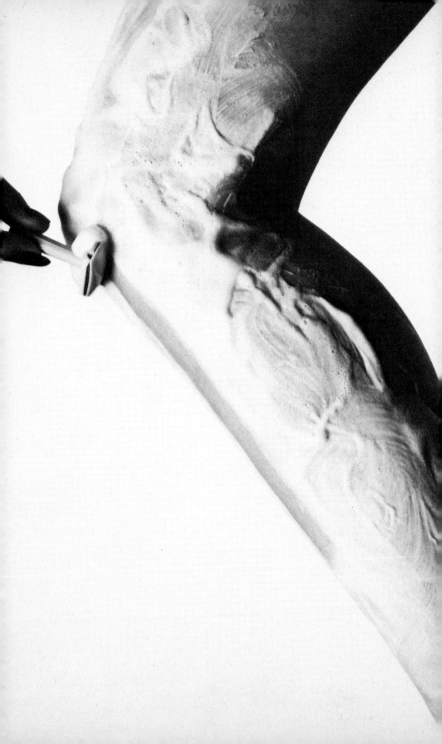

Depilation

A depilatory (a chemical normally sold as a cream, gel, powder or spray-foam) dissolves the hair shaft below the surface of the skin but doesn't destroy the root; it will sometimes weaken the hair in time, but re-growth is inevitable. There are different formulations for face and body, so make sure you buy the correct version – and, if using for the first time, try a patch test in advance and follow the directions implicitly. This method is suitable for most unwanted hair, providing the depilatory is specifically formulated for the right area.

Electrolysis

This is one of the most efficient methods and the only one offering the possibility of permanent removal, but even the best-trained technician won't guarantee there might not be some re-growth. A fine wire needle is inserted into the hair follicle and a low electric current destroys the papilla (the hair bulb) in about 40 seconds. Once the papilla is destroyed, hair from that particular bulb will never grow again. However, it is impossible to reach every papilla in an area in one session: therefore it is really only practicable for small areas (face and nipples) – legs, for instance, could take years to clear and would be extremely expensive. The pain involved varies from person to person and often depends on how close to the nerve ends the operator is working – some people just get a slight tingling sensation, others find it really hurts. But, the discomfort and expense is usually considered worth it for upper lip and chin areas and for people who are really self-conscious and distressed about an area of body hair.

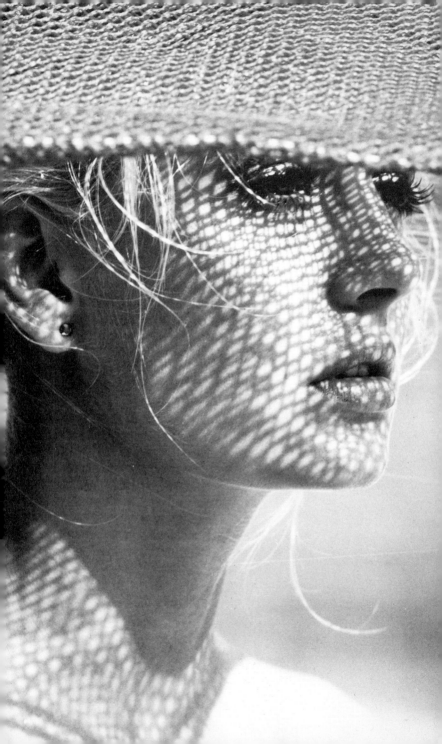

Climate:
Your Skin in the Sun and Extreme Conditions

No matter how much has been written and read about the damaging effects of the sun on skin, the world still flocks to sunny shores and slopes, and a tan is still admired . . . people are thought to look 'well' with a tan; psychologically, therefore, they feel better. And it is quite possible to have a beautiful golden tan without damaging the skin, but the skin must never be allowed to *burn*, and this takes time and discipline during the first few hours and days of summer or a sunny holiday, when the excitement of blue sky and fresh air acts like adrenalin and you tend to forget all about protection and throw caution to the winds.

The fact is, the effects of too much sun on unprotected skin will sooner or later begin to show – the natural ageing process is speeded up, the skin becomes irrevocably dehydrated, looks tough and lined like leather. And, severe over-exposure can lead to heatstroke and skin cancer. So, whether you live in the sun all the time or whether you are exposed to it once or twice a year, protection is essential if you are to prolong the beauty of your skin and have the radiance that comes from a healthy tan.

Burning is caused by ultra-violet rays stimulating the pigment-bearing cells under the epidermis into producing the brown pigment called melanin. Only the shortest of these ultra-violet rays have the strength to penetrate these cells, and it will take a day or two for this action to come to the surface and produce a change of colour. This kind of tan lasts the longest. The rays with longer waves work on melanin granules already nearing the surface and turn them dark-brown. This tan lasts less time (tans don't fade, they flake off with the dead cells). The only way to prolong a tan is to slow down the natural process of shedding dead cells: moisturizing lotions and bath oils help, or the use of a self-tanning lotion (the newest ones are combined with an after-sun moisturizer). When you burn, a scorched redness will show on the skin two or three hours after exposure – because the tiny blood-vessels on the skin's surface have dilated. The next stage, depending on the severity of the burn, is for the skin to become pimply and blistered. Once the skin is burned, however lightly, peeling of the outer, damaged layer is inevitable sooner or later. Some parts of the body are particularly vulnerable – the nose and knees, for instance, because they protrude, the back of the neck and knees, because the skin there is very tender. And, if you sunbathe nude, the breasts and genitalia, of course, are the most sensitive of all.

If you want to acquire the kind of tan that is good for you and makes you glow with health, then you must have patience and protection. If you are in the sun for the first time for many months, take it slowly – avoid the midday glare completely and sunbathe for half an hour in the morning and late in the afternoon. Increase this time each day, but still avoid the hottest part and don't be misled into thinking a cool breeze off the hills or sea has taken the sting out of the sun – it is only disguising the burning rays and you still need protection. You also need protection on the water, in the water and out of the water. It's no good putting on a sunscreen first thing in the morning and believing you are safe for the day – a lot will be lost in natural perspiration, a lot more in the water and more as you dry yourself in the sun or with a towel. You must keep reapplying a sunscreen on your face and body.

Another frequent pitfall is a skiing or mountain holiday. Like sand and water, snow reflects the powerful damaging rays, and the skin can get just as burned on what seems to be a dull or hazy day as in brilliant sunshine.

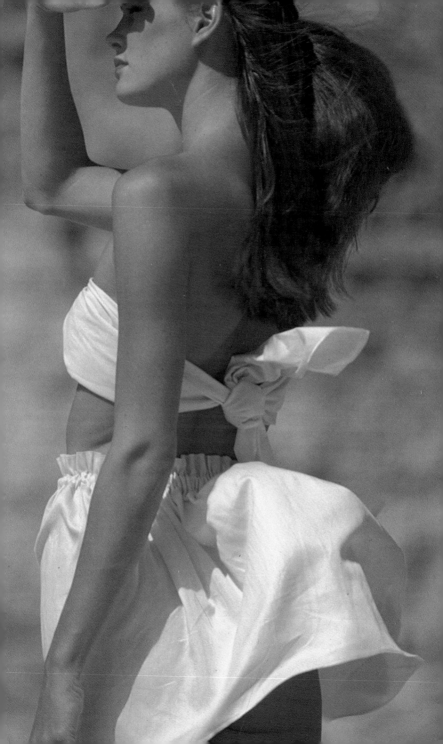

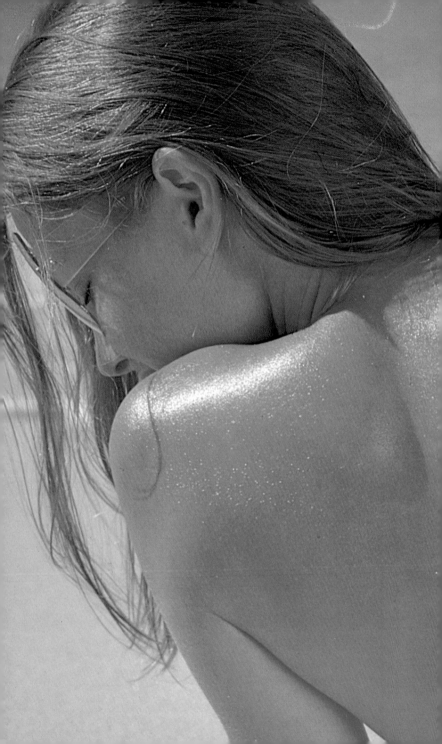

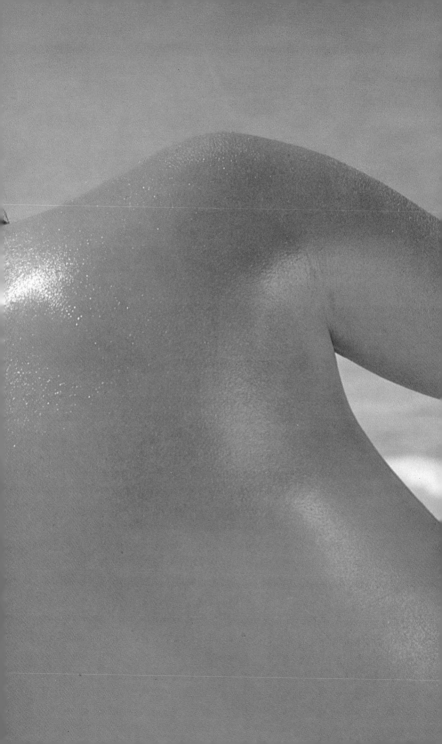

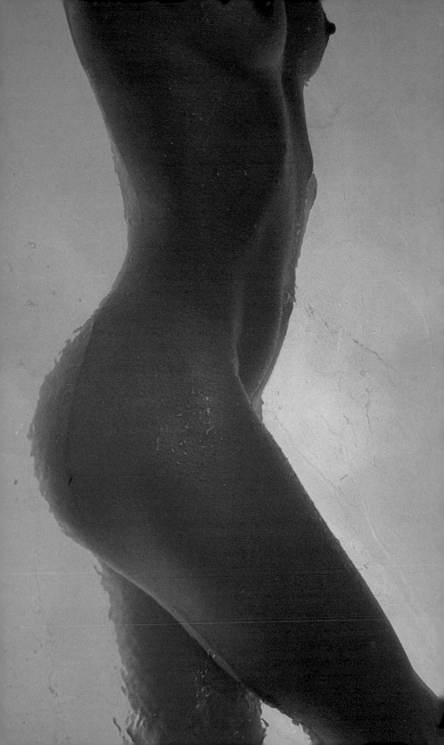

Some skins obviously burn more easily than others, but every skin needs protection to stop it from dehydrating. Very fair skin lacking in melanin will never tan deeply and red-heads with freckles just get more freckles more closely packed together. Fair skins burn quickly and take time to build a tan. Warmer-toned skins of the olive variety will be able to take more sun before burning. Brown and black skins can take even more exposure. But all skins become dryer in the sun if they are not moisturized and protected.

What to Use for Protection

Modern products range from maximum protection – sun blocks that are what they say: they block out all the rays and prevent any change of colour – to lotions, creams, gels and oils with a Sun Protective Factor (SPF) on them. To find out how long you can safely stay in the sun, you multiply the length of time it takes for your skin to burn by the SPF, e.g. if you can sunbathe five minutes before burning and you use a cream with SPF 4, you can stay in the sun safely for up to 20 minutes. If you prefer the shine of an oil to the matt absorption of a lotion or cream, be sure you choose one with a high protective ingredient; otherwise an oil is just a lubricant and provides little or no protection and will fry your precious skin. It is also wise to use a higher protective product on your face and vulnerable spots than you choose for the rest of your body. If you like to wear make-up, look for the products – foundations, lipsticks – that contain a sunscreen, and waterproof eye make-up and mascaras. The minimum looks prettiest in the sun and on a tan during the day (usually mascara and lip gloss is enough) and products with shine (frosted eyeshadows, lipsticks and blushers) look well in the evening.

Faking a Tan

The best way to have a tan and look after your skin at the same time is to use a self-tanning product that stains the skin. These are improving all the time and, although they still need careful application so you don't get a streaky effect, this temporary staining can be very satisfactory. For best results get a friend to help you achieve an even tone and the shade you want. Some beauty salons apply a tanning treatment which lasts several days and is an excellent start to a holiday; it stops you feeling white and conspicuous and therefore being so impatient to lie in the sun that you run the risk of burning.

Sun-lamps are also good but need to be used with caution – you can burn just as badly from this artificial sunshine as from the real thing. Over a period of time, however, they prepare your skin for a sunny holiday – and will prolong that carefully acquired tan after you come home. (The latest sun *beds* claim to tan safely by filtering out the harmful rays.)

Your Skin in Extreme Climates
Travelling for most of us means more time in the sun, but extremes of cold, wind or damp need just as much consideration for the skin. In hot weather, apart from the essential sun protection discussed above, the varying types of heat may make your skin react differently.

Humidity plus air pollution. You find these conditions in large cities like New York, Rome, Tel Aviv and Tokyo. You may find your skin looks grey and dirty soon after cleansing. Your make-up fades as soon as you put it on and your skin may erupt for the first time in its life. Cities like these tend to suffer from air pollution as well as humidity in summer – and pollution constantly deposits soot and grime on the skin, demanding frequent cleansing. Use a moisturizer as a barrier between your skin and the environment; you may need to choose one for an oilier skin type than you use normally in order to keep your make-up matte and stop it from disappearing. And pack something to relieve spots, should they suddenly appear. Plus sun care, of course.

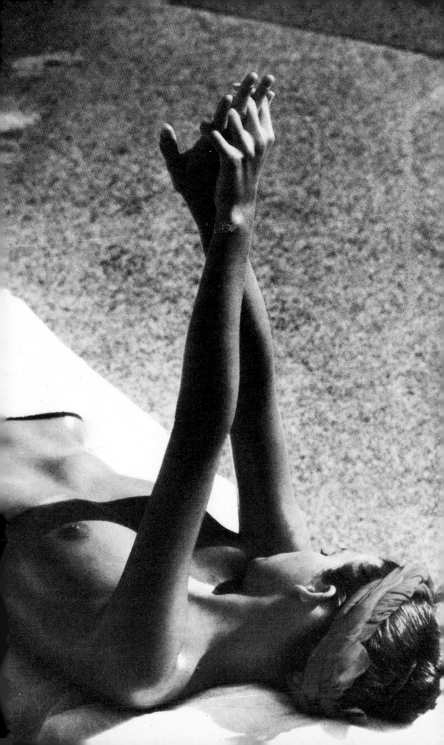

Extreme heat and aridity. Exotic spots like Marrakesh and the Nile are where you'll find this climate, and this is when skin may become extremely dry – or drier than ever before – lips parched and cracked and make-up almost impossible to apply. Take a lip emollient, a rich moisturizer for under make-up and a skin food for night-time care. Plus sun care, of course.

Tropical heat and humidity. Far-flung shores like the Seychelles, Sri Lanka and Bangkok are places to expect this climate. Skin may become excessively oily, make-up melts and hair goes limp. Keep skin extra-clean, take a good toning lotion (to refresh and tighten the texture), something to soothe spots and a moisturizer for under make-up specially formulated for oily skins (to help make-up stay put). Plus sun care, of course.

Harsh wind and extreme cold. Winter resorts such as Zermatt, Courchevel, Zurs, where high-altitude skiing is the sport, and all Polar areas are where you'll find this climate, with your skin feeling tight and dry. Use extra-rich moisturizers as well as your sun care, and avoid coming in from the intense cold and thawing out too quickly by a blazing fire – this can lead to a rupturing of the fine blood-vessels and will eventually leave red, spidery marks. Chapped skin is not a disaster and can be rehydrated with moisturizer; it usually comes from wind and is difficult to prevent if you're not going to use a thick, obvious layer of oily cream. Keep arms and legs well-lubricated too.

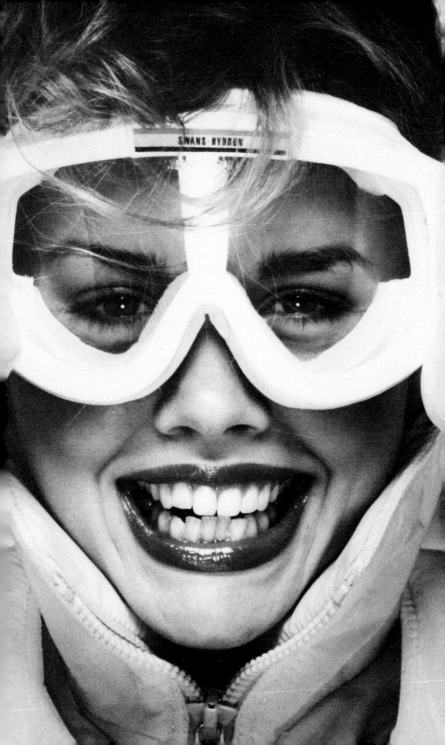

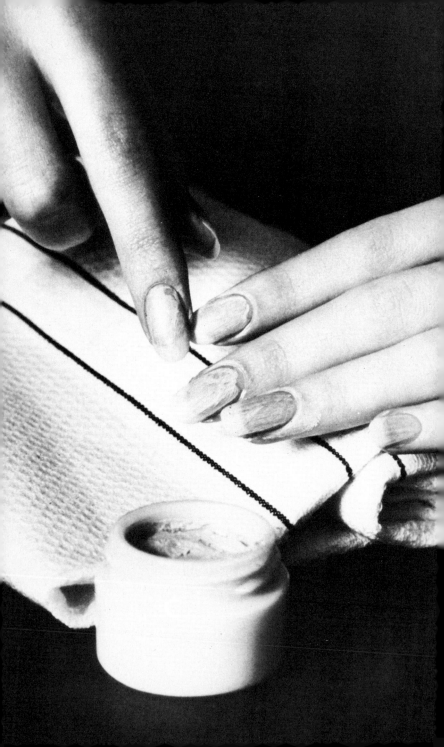

Extremities:
How to Care for Your Hands and Feet

The skin on the back of hands is fine and soft with both sebaceous and sweat-gland openings, while the skin on the palm is coarser and tougher and is one of the driest parts of the body because, unlike most other areas, it has no sebaceous glands. It does, however, have numerous sweat-glands which are often triggered off by a nervous or emotional reaction – hence the description clammy or sweaty palms – and the same is true of the soles of the feet.

Hand and wrist have great mobility from twenty-eight beautifully balanced bones. There are twenty-six bones in each foot; their strength, combined with a mass of ligaments and muscles, bears the brunt of the body weight and makes the human vertical position possible. The big toe is vital to this strength and balance as is the ball of the foot and the arch which absorbs most of the weight.

A hand can show age more quickly than any other area and, whereas surgical lifts are possible almost anywhere else, so far they have not proved successful on hands – so maintenance through care is essential. Hands that are frequently immersed in water and exposed to detergents and shampoos will dry out first. Wear rubber gloves whenever possible, always dry thoroughly and always use a hand cream afterwards. Don't neglect feet either – massage them with a good hand or body cream, paying special attention to heels and toes. Pay a regular visit to a chiropodist who will attend to patches of dry skin, corns and check for infections like athlete's foot and veruccas. This is an investment that will pay dividends by avoiding problem feet.

Manicures and pedicures are more a cosmetic treatment designed to beautify the nails, but they also keep the nail and cuticle area healthy and strong. Professional treatments are best, but you can learn to be very professional yourself and maintain finger- and toe-nails between visits. Circulation in both hands and feet is vital to their health and mobility. Here are some exercises designed to make hands more flexible and graceful, to strengthen feet and to improve circulation.

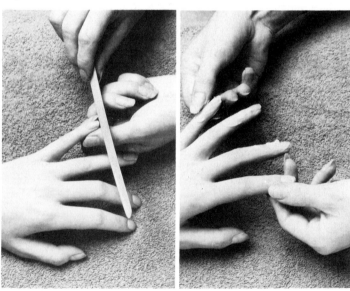

Step-by-Step Manicure
1. *File sides of the nails very gently; the ideal shape is a rounded one with straight sides. Keeping sides straight helps nails resist splitting and cracking.*
2. *Massage cuticle cream into nailbed and fingers and soak cuticles in warm water for a minute or two.*

Hand and Finger Exercises

1. Clench the fist tightly, hold a second, throw open the fingers as wide and stretched as possible. Exercise both hands simultaneously. Repeat six times.

2. Put hands straight in front of you, palms down, fingers pressed tightly against each other. Spring fingers apart as wide as possible. Repeat six times.

3. With limp, relaxed hands rotate them from the wrist in circles, first clockwise, then anti-clockwise. Turn ten circles in each direction with each hand.

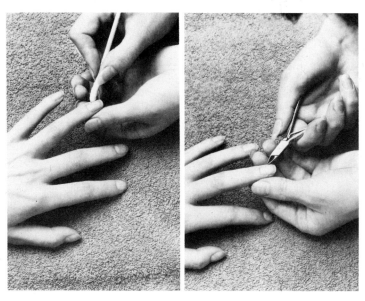

3. *Push back cuticle with orange stick wrapped in cotton wool, then with pumice stone dipped in cuticle remover (lotion).*

4. *Clip cuticle where necessary.*

73

4. Holding hands palms down, lift up slowly from the wrist, then lower, keeping the hands relaxed but not limp. Repeat ten times.

Useful Tips

A mask (the kind you use for your face) will cleanse, tone and moisturize your hands too.

A lemon will cleanse skin and bleach discoloured areas around nails. The lemon juice tends to dry the skin, so rinse off, dry and finish with a good massage of hand cream.

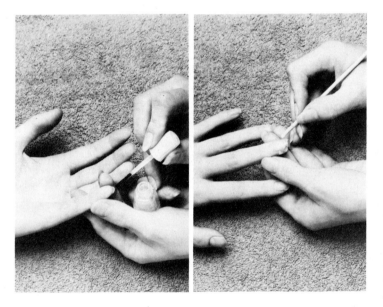

5. *Apply base coat under nail tip as well as on top of whole nail. Then wrap nail in paper nail tissue painted before wrapping with nail mender. It goes right round and under nail tip.*
6. *Prod nail tissue into place to exact shape of nail with orange stick.*

Warm olive oil is useful as a special treatment for hands, especially in winter when they are inclined to be chapped and dry. Soak them in it for about half an hour.

Cotton gloves should be worn at night whenever you can. Put them on over a layer of hand cream or petroleum jelly.

Gloves should be worn much of the time; heavy duty ones for gardening, rubber for washing activities and leather, silk or wool outside when it's cold, wet or snowing. Even in summer leather or cotton will prevent hands drying.

Patrice Casanova

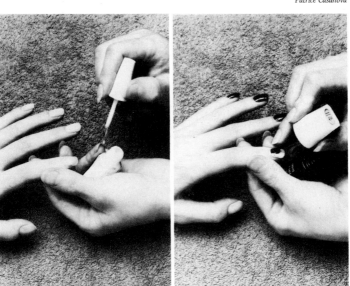

7. *Paint on another complete base coat over top of nail and tissue to seal in wrapping.*

8. *Apply an extra base coat as a top sealer which prevents polish cracking or splitting. Apply nail polish under nail tip and on top. Repeat once.*

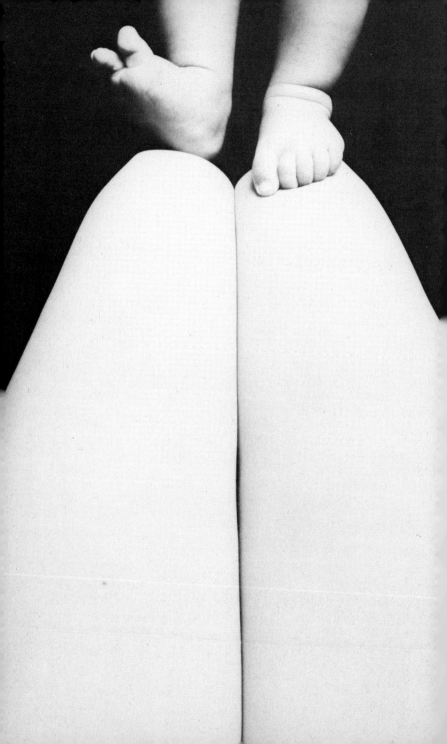

Foot Exercises

One of the best exercises of all for the feet is walking barefoot along a beach; try keeping to the water's edge, where the sand is wet. Others are:

1. Stand up straight, feet pointed ahead, and raise yourself up on your toes, then lower. This helps strengthen the foot arch and tendons around the ankle joint.

2. Cover a large book with a towel and place in front of you; with feet on book, toes extending over the edge, curl toes and try to pick up the towel. This helps strengthen the metatarsal arch, overcomes the tendency for toes to curl up and helps prevent callouses.

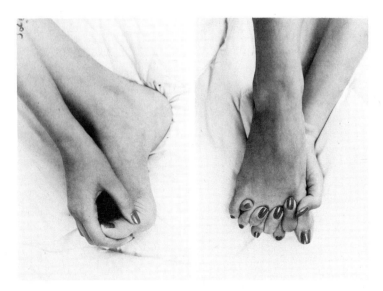

Six exercises to put you back on your feet. Spare five minutes to do them, once a day, every day.

*1. Holding your foot in one hand, twist ankle inwards, then out. Repeat with the other foot. **2.** Grab all your toes, bend them upwards and release. Take each toe separately and roll it around in a circle. **3.** Slip*

Essentials

Emery boards – for shaping nails and smoothing away hardened skin at the sides.

Pumice-stone – to soften rough cuticles or callouses and keep legs smooth.

Cuticle cream – to keep cuticles smooth and soft, avoid hangnails and encourage strong nail growth.

Orange sticks – for nudging back cuticles very gently and pushing the cuticle cream underneath.

Hand cream – to keep skin soft and supple.

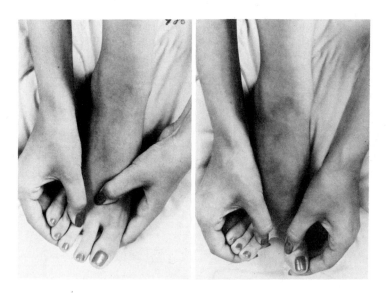

your fingers between your toes. Bend your foot down and pull it towards you. **4.** *Squeeze your foot with both hands while flexing your toes up and down. Pull each toe gently away from the one next to it.* **5.** *Press each toe firmly between thumb and index-finger, then press thumbs along the top of the foot between each of the bones at the base of the toes. Continue up to the ankle.*

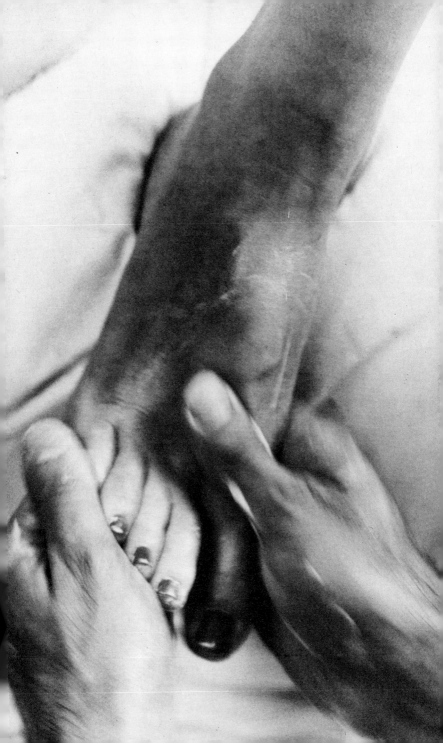

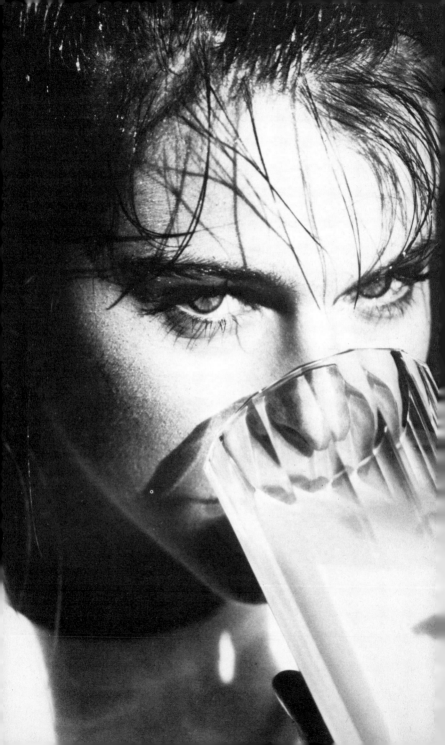

Skin Health: Eating

All skins, even healthy skins, need correct feeding and treatment, not only externally but internally. What you eat can improve or do irreparable harm to your skin. Oily skin, for example, may reflect a lack of vitamin B2 (riboflavin); this can be corrected by adding good natural food sources to your diet – liver and more milk, for instance. Oily and dimpled skin may be caused by shortage of vitamin B6 (pyridoxine). Good food sources for this include pork, veal, wheatgerm and bananas. Vitamin A is a primary skin-health vitamin and is found in dark-green and deep-yellow vegetables and fruits. Skins that are drying and ageing too soon may lack the F vitamins, pantothenic acid and niacin. Eggs and liver are excellent sources of pantothenic acid; niacin is found in beef and mushrooms.

Too much alcohol isn't good for the skin – nor is smoking. Drinking lots of water – tap or mineral – does wonders for it.

Crash diets, where the weight is removed suddenly and put back when the diet is over, are damaging to the skin and will be noticeable as you grow older, when the skin loses its elasticity and is unable to spring back. It will become flabby and lose its texture. The answer is to develop a healthy eating pattern that becomes an unbreakable habit very early in life, getting rid of any overweight gradually, so that it goes for good and the new weight is maintained. Try to avoid fatty foods, highly spiced foods, sweets, cakes, biscuits, sauces and too many rich dairy foods; learn to like fresh fruit, salads and vegetables, grilled fish and meat and wholewheat bread. A diet high in these items and water, and low in the others and alcohol, will keep your skin in good shape for a lifetime.

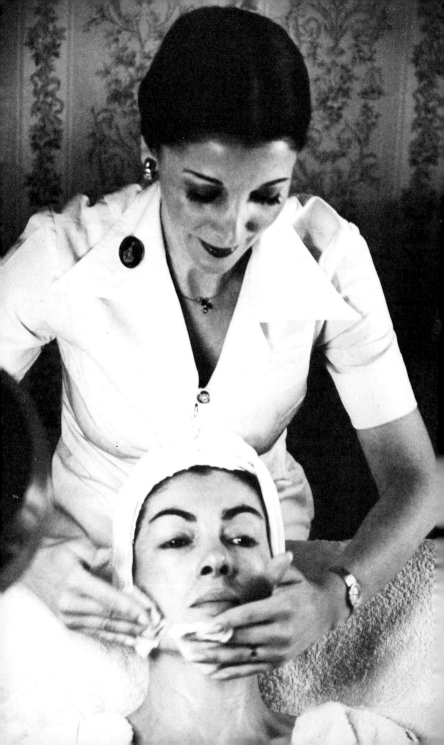

Professional Skin Treatments:
Face and Body

Professional treatments range from a cleansing facial in a beauty salon through massage and skin peeling to cosmetic plastic surgery. Considered by some as an extravagant indulgence, they can do much to help beauty both on a mostly psychological short-term basis, and in the long term, by an extension of the youthful qualities of the skin and body.

Face
Professional facials. Theories differ about the benefits of massaging the face, and it is a matter of personal opinion, but a deep-cleansing treatment can do nothing but good. Personal recommendation is a good way of finding an expert beautician, and it is important that you like the feel of their hands and get on well with them because the relaxation that should be part of the treatment is vital to the results. It is also important that the products smell and feel pleasant to you – who wants to close their eyes for twenty minutes under, what is to them, an evil-smelling mask? After a cleansing treatment it is usually recommended that no make-up is worn for a day – or twenty-four hours if possible – to give the skin a chance to breathe and make the most of its new vitality. So, make an appointment with that in mind. Facials also help to reduce wrinkles.

Wrinkles – or lines – are one of the first signs that skin is beginning to age and usually appear around the eyes or mouth, caused by premature dehydration in these delicate areas. There are new creams coming on the market all the time as a result of constant research into this problem and, although none will eliminate the lines, many of them help prevent their deepening and multiplying too fast. Professional facials often help too, with the use of special oils, emollients, massage and masks. But the only way to soften or remove them is through *peeling* – or dermabrasion. These are medical procedures carried out by doctors or highly qualified beauticians. They are an extension of cosmetic exfoliating – the removal of dead surface cells from the skin by means of an abrasive cream, gel or lotion applied with a brush or rough-textured pad. The result is better-textured skin with a more even tone. As skin grows older and lines begin to deepen, the only way to help is by literally removing the top layer of skin and revealing the new one underneath. This is done either by chemical surgery or by dermabrasion, the latter method of *planing* often being used on scars, as it can be done on small areas. Both methods take from three to six months before the final improvement is visible.

Plastic surgery is the most drastic method of improving or prolonging the youthful aspects of face and body, the cosmetic possibilities being realized after the science was pioneered during the war in rebuilding badly burned and scarred servicemen. Only carried out by highly qualified surgeons, these operations can restructure for life features like noses, ears or chins; reduce fatty areas by removing the fatty deposits from under the surface or taking part of the skin and bone away; or improving shape by adding bone or silicone. Wrinkles, lines and sagging skin are smoothed and tightened by lifting and tucking away. Successful operations are now carried out on: breasts, buttocks, chins, ears, eyes, face, neck, nose, stomach and thighs.

How long they last depends on the individual – age, inherited problems, stress and how much care is taken with diet, exercise, skin and sun care after treatment.

Body

Plastic surgery is a drastic and often expensive means of improving body shape and texture, but operations like breast enlargement are usually very rewarding. A good exercise routine, started early in life and practised regularly, can do much to improve posture and shape and keeps muscles working, so that the body is supple and graceful.

Massage is enormously beneficial to the body – the gentle, kneading strokes revitalizing muscles, decreasing tension and stimulating circulation. It is a great tranquillizer – some people actually fall asleep during the massage – and, as most masseurs use an emollient cream or oil, the skin benefits too. In conjunction with a slimming diet and exercise, massage will help get rid of overweight and reshape the body. As with beauticians, it is important to find a masseur that suits you – although the methods may be basically the same, individuals develop their own special routines, using more or less pressure, for instance, and choosing special oils for their aroma or therapeutic values.

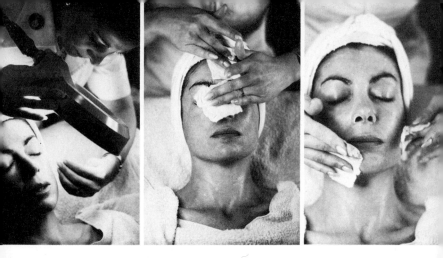

Step-by-Step Deep Cleanse Treatment

This is a professional cleansing treatment that nourishes and re-balances the skin, improving elasticity and tone, softening wrinkles. Originally conceived to help acne, it was discovered that this method, using a galvanic/high-frequency machine, was equally good for general skin care. The treatment is here undergone by the author.

1. *The skin is examined to establish its type and which products to use.* **2.** *The skin is cleansed with a suitable product: here, one for sensitive skin with broken veins.* **3.** *The skin is toned with a suitable product and the face is blotted dry with tissue.* **4.** *The skin is re-examined and blackheads and sebum removed.* **5.** *A special solution,*

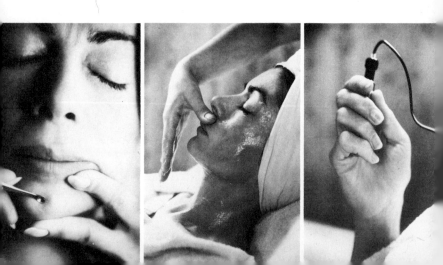

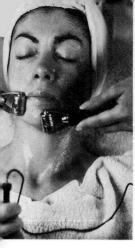
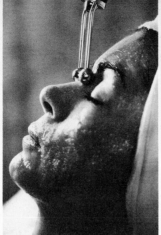
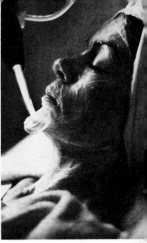

Electro Z, is used to help overcome the skin's natural resistance to electric current and catiogenic gel is smoothed over face and neck. **6.** A small metal bar is held; this makes the skin receptive to the galvanic current. The machine is switched on and the current adjusted. **7-9.** Roller applicator heads are passed over the skin's surface to loosen accumulated grease and dirt in the pores; a light perspiration is set up, which rejects the dirt. **10.** The machine is switched to high frequency and oxygen cream and gauze are spread over to boost the effect of the treatment. **11.** The face is massaged with a liquid to contract the pores, nourish and regenerate the skin. A mask is then chosen, suitable for the type of skin. **12.** The mask is cleaned off, the skin toned and moisturized. The fresh clean skin should not be made-up for twenty-four hours.

Sandra Lousada

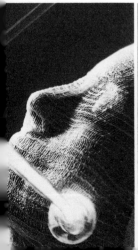
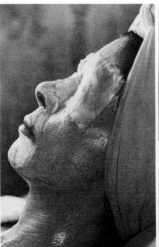
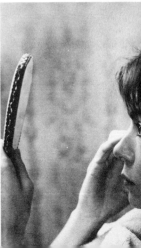

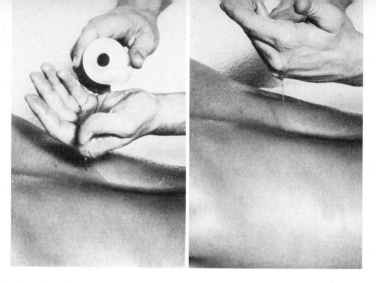

There is still nothing more effective after a hot sauna than a professional massage to revive one. One of the oldest methods, although little practised in Europe, is the Shiatsu – an extremely relaxing technique of applying pressure to one's nerve endings, which automatically releases all muscular pain, stress and tension.

An added bonus with massage, by traditional or modern methods, is the dislodging of fat cells. By stimulating circulation it disperses fatty deposits and rejuvenates the skin.

The photographs show the masseur concentrating on the area of the back that causes most trouble.

Renato Grignaschi

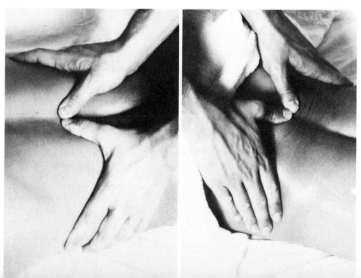

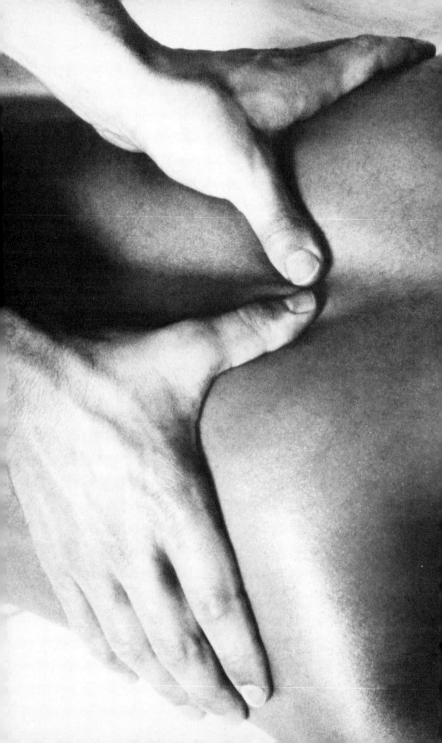

Index

MORE ABOUT PENGUINS
AND PELICANS

For further information about books available from Penguins please write to Dept EP, Penguin Books Ltd, Harmondsworth, Middlesex UB7 ODA.

In the U.S.A.: For a complete list of books available from Penguins in the United States write to Dept CS, Penguin Books, 625 Madison Avenue, New York, New York 10022.

In Canada: For a complete list of books available from Penguins in Canada write to Penguin Books Canada Ltd, 2801 John Street, Markham, Ontario L3R 1B4.

In Australia: For a complete list of books available from Penguins in Australia write to the Marketing Department, Penguin Books Australia Ltd, P.O. Box 257, Ringwood, Victoria 3134.

In New Zealand: For a complete list of books available from Penguins in New Zealand write to the Marketing Department, Penguin Books (NZ) Ltd, P.O. Box 4019, Auckland 10.

VOGUE GUIDE TO HAIR CARE

The book for everyone who wants glossy, healthy hair! Here you can find out about your hair's structure and type, what happens to it with age, and how to look after it. The author advises you on finding a style to suit you and to keep you looking your best – whatever the weather. There is detailed advice on colouring with natural and man-made dyes, on permanent waving and straightening, and on styles for special occasions, wigs and hairpieces. And, as diet affects hair, the guide includes useful recipes, an A–Z of hair care, plus an illustrated glossary of recent cuts and styles.

VOGUE GUIDE TO MAKE-UP

Your make-up routine and the equipment you'll need is detailed for you here, whatever your colouring or skin type, whatever the lighting, climate or time of day. Here are illustrations with expert advice to show you how to do it, plus notes on what to wear with what, how to make the most of your best features and guidelines for the different age-groups. There's also an A–Z of scent terms and, to add the final polish, twelve steps to a professional pedicure, tips on how to choose your nail colour and how to varnish your nails.

Also in Penguin by Bronwen Meredith

VOGUE BODY AND BEAUTY BOOK

VOGUE NATURAL HEALTH AND BEAUTY